LYMPHOMA DIET COOKBOOK

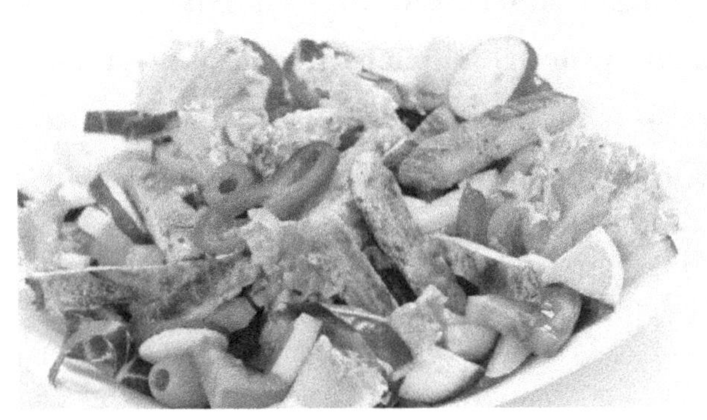

Unlocking Wellness Through Immune Boosting Meals to Support Lymphoma Management and Recovery to Enjoy Healthy Living

PATRICIA R. TARRANT

CONTENTS

INTRODUCTION

Sarah, after being diagnosed with lymphoma, went on a path of healing through a carefully personalized diet. She adopted a holistic approach to her health, guided by a lymphoma diet cookbook. The cookbook, which was filled with nutrient-rich meals and expert advice, became her compass as she faced the trials of cancer.

Sarah's diet was high in anti-inflammatory foods and antioxidants, as well as immune-boosting minerals. In her meals, she included a range of colorful fruits and vegetables, nutritious grains, lean proteins, and healthy fats. Her culinary adventure included experimenting with anti-cancer herbs and spices to enhance both flavor and health effects.

Sarah came a step closer to recovery with each meal, realizing the enormous impact nutrition may have on her body's ability to fight cancer. She faithfully followed the cookbook's instructions, learning to make informed decisions that aided her immune system and overall vigor.

Her journey was not without difficulties. Sarah struggled with uncertainty and discouragement, but the incremental improvement in her health kept her going. Her dietary efforts were supplemented by regular contact with healthcare professionals, ensuring a complete approach to lymphoma management.

Sarah's dedication to the lymphoma diet paid off over time. Her energy levels climbed, and the treatment's adverse effects became more manageable. Medical evaluations indicated favorable results, confirming the effectiveness of a lymphoma-specific diet.

Sarah's tale became an uplifting example of the power of lifestyle modifications in managing and even curing health issues. Her accomplishment not only emphasized the importance of nutrition in cancer care, but also the value of an individualized approach led by a credible resource like the lymphoma diet cookbook.

Sarah not only beat cancer, but she also gained a new awareness for the role of nutrition in overall health. Her tale became a beacon of hope for others facing similar issues, inspiring them to investigate the transformational potential of a well-balanced diet.

Welcome to "Lymphoma Diet Cookbook," a culinary guide to help people achieve well-being while controlling cancer. This cookbook goes beyond recipes, providing a complete dietary plan designed exclusively for persons dealing with lymphoma.

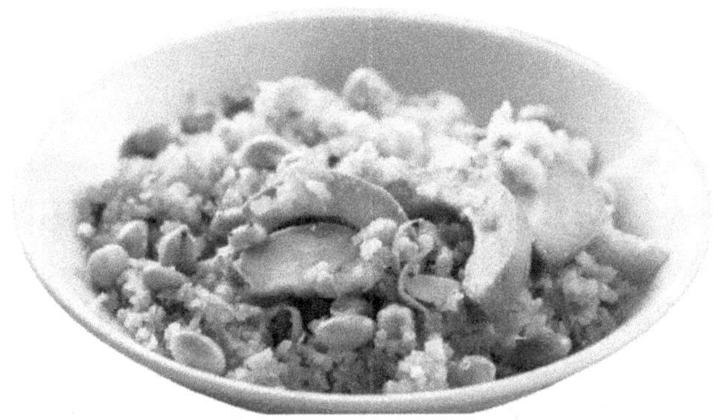

"I am resilient, and my spirit is stronger than any challenge I face with lymphoma."

"Every day, my body is getting stronger, and I am moving towards healing."

CHAPTER 1: UNDERSTANDING LYMPHOMA

Lymphoma is a cancer that starts in the lymphatic system, which is an important part of the immune system. Lymph nodes, the spleen, the thymus gland, and bone marrow are all part of the lymphatic system. Lymphoma develops when aberrant lymphocytes, a kind of white blood cell, proliferate uncontrolled, resulting in tumor growth.

Lymphoma is classified into two types: Hodgkin lymphoma (HL) and non-Hodgkin lymphoma (NHL). The presence of Reed-Sternberg cells distinguishes Hodgkin lymphoma from non-Hodgkin lymphoma, which covers a varied range of lymphomas with various subtypes.

Lymphoma causes and risk factors are unknown, but certain risk factors may enhance the likelihood of having the disease. A compromised immune system, exposure to certain viruses (such as the Epstein-Barr virus), a family history of lymphoma, and certain autoimmune illnesses are also risk factors.

Swollen lymph nodes, unexplained weight loss, exhaustion, night sweats, and itching are all common signs of lymphoma. These symptoms, however, can be connected with a variety of illnesses, emphasizing the significance of getting medical assistance for an appropriate diagnosis.

Lymphoma is diagnosed using a combination of medical history analysis, physical examination, imaging testing (CT scans, PET scans), and lymph node biopsy. A biopsy can assist define the kind and subtype of lymphoma, which is important for developing an effective treatment approach.

IMPORTANCE OF NUTRITION IN LYMPHOMA MANAGEMENT

Nutrition is critical in the treatment of lymphoma, a malignancy that affects the lymphatic system. Individuals receiving treatment can benefit significantly from a well-balanced and nutrient-rich diet, which can assist to promote overall health, manage side effects, and improve the body's ability to fight the disease.

1. Immune Function Support: A healthy diet is vital for keeping a strong immune system. A compromised immune system is commonly a worry for people with lymphoma, due to both the disease and the therapies. Proper nutrition can help strengthen the immune response, boosting the body's natural defense against cancer cells.

2. Managing Treatment Side Effects: Lymphoma therapies, such as chemotherapy and radiation therapy, can cause nausea, exhaustion, and weight loss. A well-planned diet can help with these symptoms. To prevent nausea and preserve energy levels, for example, easily digestible, nutrient-dense foods may be recommended.

3. Maintaining Weight and Muscle Mass: It is critical to maintain a healthy weight during cancer treatment. Adequate protein intake is especially crucial for preventing muscle atrophy and promoting tissue regeneration. To assist clients in maintaining their nutritional status, this lymphoma diet cookbook features recipes that focus on high-protein, calorie-dense meals.

4. Managing Nutrient Deficiencies: Cancer and its therapies can occasionally result in nutrient deficiencies. This lymphoma diet cookbook stresses on foods high in important vitamins and minerals, which can assist to compensate for any deficits that may occur. This involves consuming a wide range of fruits, vegetables, and whole grains.

5. Reducing Inflammation: Chronic inflammation has been linked to the development and progression of cancer. Certain foods have anti-inflammatory capabilities, therefore this lymphoma diet cookbook includes recipes with anti-inflammatory elements including fatty fish, turmeric, and leafy greens.

6. Hydration and Detoxification: Staying hydrated is essential for overall health and is especially important during cancer treatment, as it supports kidney function and aids in the removal of toxins from the body. This lymphoma diet cookbook recommends hydrating beverages and water-rich foods.

FOODS TO EAT AND FOODS TO AVOID

A lymphoma diet is making conscious dietary choices to enhance general health and manage the condition.

Here are some general tips for lymphoma diet foods to include and avoid:

Foods to Include:

1. Lean Proteins: Choose lean protein sources such as poultry, fish, lentils, and tofu. Protein is necessary for muscle mass maintenance, immune function support, and tissue repair.

2. Colorful Fruits and Vegetables: Include a range of antioxidant-rich fruits and vegetables, as well as vitamins and minerals. These can aid in the fight against oxidative stress, inflammation, and overall wellness. Berries, leafy greens, and cruciferous veggies are all fantastic options.

3. Whole Grains: Choose whole grains such as brown rice, quinoa, oats, and whole wheat. These grains contain fiber, important nutrients, and a constant flow of energy, which aids digestion and prevents blood sugar spikes.

4. Healthy Fats: Avocados, almonds, seeds, and olive oil are all good sources of healthful fats. These fats supply necessary fatty acids and can aid in the reduction of inflammation in the body.

5. Hydrating Beverages: Stay hydrated by drinking water, herbal teas, and broths. Hydration is essential for general health and can aid in the management of probable medication adverse effects such as nausea and exhaustion.

6. Probiotics: Include probiotic-rich foods such as yogurt, kefir, and fermented vegetables in your diet. Probiotics promote intestinal health, which is necessary for immune function and nutritional absorption.

7. Herbs and spices: Use anti-inflammatory and immune-boosting herbs and spices such as turmeric, ginger, and garlic. These can add flavor to foods while also potentially delivering health advantages.

Foods to Avoid:

1. Processed Foods: Limit your consumption of highly processed foods, which often contain additives, preservatives, and harmful fats.

Processed foods can cause inflammation and deplete critical nutrients.

2. Sugary Foods and Beverages: Limit your intake of sugary foods and beverages, as too much sugar might impair immune function and lead to inflammation. Instead of sugary snacks, choose entire fruits.

3. High-Fat and Fried Foods: Limit your consumption of high-fat and fried foods, which can be difficult to digest and may contribute to weight gain. Consider using healthier cooking methods such as grilling, baking, or steaming.

4. Red and Processed Meats: Red and processed meats should be avoided since they have been linked to an increased risk of some malignancies. Choose lean proteins such as fish, chicken, and plant-based alternatives.

5. Excessive Dairy: Some people may find that limiting their dairy intake helps them manage symptoms such as bloating or digestive pain. Experiment with dairy substitutes such as almond or soy milk.

6. Alcohol: Limit your alcohol usage because it can interfere with certain medications and damage your immune system. If alcohol is consumed, it should be drunk in moderation and discussed with healthcare providers.

7. High-Sodium Foods: Limit your intake of high-sodium foods, as too much salt can cause fluid retention and high blood pressure. Instead of salt, choose fresh, healthy foods and season dishes with herbs and spices.

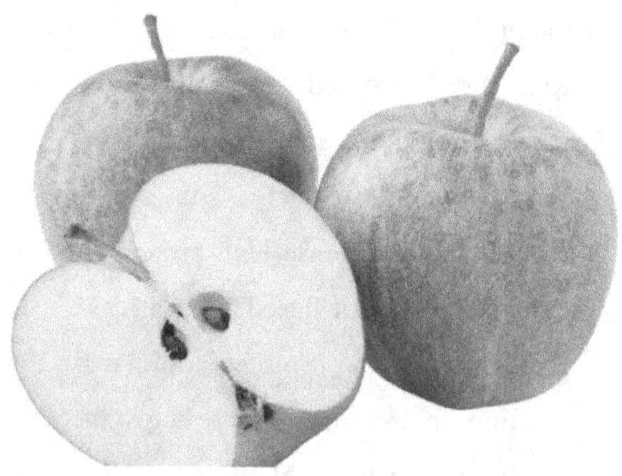

CHAPTER 2: LYMPHOMA DIET SHOPPING LIST

Here's a grocery list for a Lymphoma-friendly diet that emphasizes nutrient-dense, anti-inflammatory foods:

Proteins:

- Lean poultry (chicken, turkey)
- Fish (salmon, trout, mackerel)
- Legumes (beans, lentils)
- Tofu or tempeh

Vegetables:

- Leafy greens (spinach, kale, collard greens)
- Cruciferous vegetables (broccoli, cauliflower, Brussels sprouts)
- Colorful vegetables (carrots, bell peppers, tomatoes)
- Garlic and onions for flavor and potential anti-inflammatory benefits

Fruits:

- Berries (blueberries, strawberries, raspberries)

- Citrus fruits (oranges, grapefruits)
- Apples and pears
- Avocado for healthy fats

Whole Grains:
- Quinoa
- Brown rice
- Whole wheat or whole grain bread
- Oats

Healthy Fats:
- Olive oil
- Nuts (almonds, walnuts)
- Seeds (flaxseeds, chia seeds)
- Fatty fish (salmon, mackerel)

Dairy or Dairy Alternatives:
- Low-fat or Greek yogurt
- Almond or coconut milk

Herbs and Spices:
- Turmeric
- Ginger

- Basil, thyme, rosemary for seasoning without added salt

Beverages:
- Green tea
- Water with lemon or cucumber for hydration

Snacks:
- Hummus with vegetable sticks
- Air-popped popcorn
- Fresh fruit slices

Avoid or Limit:
- Processed and red meats
- Refined sugars and sweets
- High-fat dairy
- Excessive salt and processed foods

EATING OUT ON THE LYMPHOMA DIET

Eating out when battling cancer necessitates careful planning to guarantee a well-balanced and nutritionally supporting meal.

When dining out, keep the following considerations in mind:

1. Select Restaurants Wisely: Look for restaurants that offer a wide range of menu selections, including fresh and whole meals. Many places now include nutritional information, which can assist you in making informed decisions.

2. Prioritize Lean Proteins: Choose foods with lean protein sources such grilled chicken, fish, or lentils. These proteins are required for muscle mass preservation following lymphoma treatment.

3. Fruits and vegetables should be highlighted: Look for dishes that contain a variety of colorful fruits and vegetables. These contain antioxidants and important elements that are beneficial to overall wellness.

4. Choose Whole Grains: When available, choose whole grain options such as whole wheat bread or brown rice. These give fiber as well as long-lasting energy.

5. Mindful Portion Control: To avoid overeating, be mindful of portion amounts. If available, consider splitting dishes or ordering half quantities.

6. Customize Your Order: Feel free to modify your order to match your dietary requirements. To make your meal more lymphoma-friendly, ask for sauces and dressings on the side, as well as substitutes.

7. Limit Processed and Fried Foods: Limit your consumption of processed and fried foods, which may contribute to inflammation. Instead, choose grilled, steaming, or baked choices.

8. Stay Hydrated: To stay hydrated, drink water or other low-calorie, non-sweetened liquids. Sugary drinks and alcohol should be avoided because they can raise blood sugar levels.

9. Consider Dietary Restrictions: If you have any dietary restrictions or intolerances, make sure the restaurant staff is aware of them. Many businesses can meet unusual demands.

10. Sugars and Desserts Should Be Consumed in Moderation: Desserts and sugary snacks should be consumed in moderation. Consider fresh fruit or sharing a dessert with friends to fulfill your sweet desire without consuming too much sugar.

11. Request Professional Guidance: If you're unsure about your menu options, don't be afraid to ask the server for recommendations or changes depending on your dietary preferences and health needs.

12. Take Your Time While Eating: Eat gently and thoroughly. This not only improves the meal experience, but also allows your body more time to recognize when you're full.

7-DAY MEAL PLAN

Day 1:

Breakfast: Quinoa Breakfast Bowl (quinoa, mixed berries, sliced almonds, honey)

Ingredients:

- 1 cup quinoa
- 2 cups water
- 1 cup mixed berries (strawberries, blueberries, raspberries)
- 1/4 cup sliced almonds
- 2 tablespoons honey

Instructions:

1. Rinse the quinoa under cold water to remove any bitterness.
2. In a medium saucepan, combine the rinsed quinoa and water. Bring it to a boil, then reduce the heat to low, cover, and simmer for 15 minutes or until the quinoa is cooked and water is absorbed.

3. While the quinoa is cooking, wash the mixed berries and slice any larger berries into bite-sized pieces.

4. Once the quinoa is cooked, fluff it with a fork and let it cool slightly.

5. In a serving bowl, layer the cooked quinoa, mixed berries, and sliced almonds.

6. Drizzle the honey over the top of the bowl.

7. Gently toss the ingredients together to combine and evenly distribute the flavors.

8. Serve the quinoa breakfast bowl warm and enjoy a wholesome, nutritious start to your day!

Lunch: Lentil and Vegetable Soup with Whole Grain Roll

Ingredients:

- 1 cup dry green or brown lentils, rinsed and drained
- 1 onion, finely chopped
- 2 carrots, diced
- 2 celery stalks, chopped
- 3 cloves garlic, minced
- 1 can (14 oz) diced tomatoes
- 6 cups vegetable broth

- 1 teaspoon ground cumin
- 1 teaspoon ground coriander
- 1 teaspoon dried thyme
- Salt and pepper to taste
- 2 cups kale, chopped
- 1 tablespoon olive oil
- Fresh parsley for garnish

For Whole Grain Rolls:

- 4 whole grain rolls

Instructions:

1. In a large pot, heat olive oil over medium heat. Add chopped onions, carrots, and celery. Sauté until vegetables are softened, about 5 minutes.
2. Add minced garlic, cumin, coriander, and thyme to the pot. Stir well to coat the vegetables in the spices.
3. Pour in the vegetable broth, diced tomatoes (with their juice), and rinsed lentils. Season with salt and pepper to taste. Bring the soup to a boil, then reduce the heat to low, cover, and simmer for 25-30 minutes or until lentils are tender.

4. While the soup is simmering, preheat the oven for the whole grain rolls according to the package instructions. Bake the rolls until golden brown.

5. Add chopped kale to the soup during the last 10 minutes of cooking, allowing it to wilt and cook through.

6. Taste the soup and adjust the seasoning if needed. Remove the pot from heat.

7. Ladle the lentil and vegetable soup into bowls and garnish with fresh parsley.

8. Serve the soup hot with a side of whole grain rolls.

Dinner: Grilled Chicken Salad (mixed greens, cherry tomatoes, cucumber, grilled chicken, light vinaigrette)

Ingredients:

For the Salad:

- 2 boneless, skinless chicken breasts
- Salt and pepper to taste
- 8 cups mixed salad greens (lettuce, spinach, arugula, etc.)

- 1 cup cherry tomatoes, halved
- 1 cucumber, sliced
- 1/4 cup red onion, thinly sliced

For the Grilled Chicken Marinade:

- 2 tablespoons olive oil
- 2 tablespoons balsamic vinegar
- 2 cloves garlic, minced
- 1 teaspoon dried oregano
- Salt and pepper to taste

For the Light Vinaigrette:

- 3 tablespoons extra-virgin olive oil
- 1 tablespoon balsamic vinegar
- 1 teaspoon Dijon mustard
- 1 teaspoon honey
- Salt and pepper to taste

Instructions:

1. In a bowl, mix the ingredients for the grilled chicken marinade: olive oil, balsamic vinegar, minced garlic, dried oregano, salt, and pepper. Place the chicken breasts in a zip-top bag and pour the marinade over them. Seal the bag and refrigerate for at least 30 minutes.

2. Preheat the grill to medium-high heat. Grill the marinated chicken breasts for about 6-8 minutes per side or until fully cooked. Allow the chicken to rest for a few minutes before slicing it into thin strips.

3. In a large salad bowl, combine the mixed salad greens, cherry tomatoes, sliced cucumber, and red onion.

4. For the light vinaigrette, whisk together the extra-virgin olive oil, balsamic vinegar, Dijon mustard, honey, salt, and pepper in a small bowl.

5. Drizzle the light vinaigrette over the salad and toss gently to coat the greens evenly.

6. Arrange the grilled chicken strips on top of the salad.

7. Serve the grilled chicken salad immediately, offering additional vinaigrette on the side if desired.

Snack: Greek Yogurt with Berries

Ingredients:

- 1 cup Greek yogurt
- 1/2 cup mixed berries (strawberries, blueberries, raspberries)

- 1 tablespoon honey

- 2 tablespoons chopped nuts (almonds, walnuts, or pistachios)

- Fresh mint leaves for garnish (optional)

Instructions:

1. Spoon the Greek yogurt into a serving bowl or individual containers.

2. Wash the mixed berries and pat them dry with a paper towel.

3. Arrange the mixed berries on top of the Greek yogurt.

4. Drizzle honey over the yogurt and berries for sweetness.

5. Sprinkle the chopped nuts over the top for added crunch and flavor.

6. If desired, garnish the yogurt with fresh mint leaves for a burst of freshness.

7. Serve the Greek yogurt with berries immediately and enjoy a delightful and nutritious snack or breakfast.

Day 2:

Breakfast: Avocado Toast with Smoked Salmon on Whole Grain Bread

Ingredients:

- 2 slices of whole grain bread
- 1 ripe avocado
- 1 tablespoon lemon juice
- Salt and pepper to taste
- 4 ounces smoked salmon
- Red onion, thinly sliced (optional)
- Capers for garnish (optional)
- Fresh dill for garnish (optional)

Instructions:

1. Toast the whole grain bread slices to your desired level of crispiness.
2. While the bread is toasting, cut the ripe avocado in half, remove the pit, and scoop the flesh into a bowl.
3. Mash the avocado with a fork, and then add lemon juice, salt, and pepper to taste. Mix well.
4. Once the bread is toasted, spread the mashed avocado evenly over each slice.

5. Lay slices of smoked salmon on top of the mashed avocado.

6. If desired, add thinly sliced red onion on top of the smoked salmon.

7. Garnish with capers and fresh dill for added flavor.

8. Serve the avocado toast with smoked salmon immediately and enjoy a delicious and nutritious meal.

Lunch: Chickpea and Spinach Salad (chickpeas, spinach, cherry tomatoes, lemon-tahini dressing)

Ingredients:
For the Salad:

- 2 cans (15 oz each) chickpeas, drained and rinsed
- 5 cups fresh spinach, washed and chopped
- 1 cup cherry tomatoes, halved

For the Lemon-Tahini Dressing:

- 1/4 cup tahini
- 3 tablespoons fresh lemon juice
- 2 tablespoons olive oil

- 1 clove garlic, minced
- 1 teaspoon honey
- Salt and pepper to taste
- 2 tablespoons water (optional, to thin the dressing)

Instructions:

1. In a large salad bowl, combine the chickpeas, chopped fresh spinach, and halved cherry tomatoes.
2. In a separate bowl, whisk together the tahini, fresh lemon juice, olive oil, minced garlic, honey, salt, and pepper to create the dressing.
3. If the dressing is too thick, you can add water, one tablespoon at a time, until you reach your desired consistency.
4. Pour the lemon-tahini dressing over the chickpea and spinach mixture. Toss gently to coat the salad evenly.
5. Allow the salad to marinate in the dressing for a few minutes to enhance the flavors.
6. Taste the salad and adjust the seasoning if necessary.
7. Serve the chickpea and spinach salad immediately, or refrigerate for later use.

Dinner: Baked Cod with Lemon Dill Sauce, Quinoa Pilaf, Steamed Broccoli

Ingredients:

For Baked Cod:

- 4 cod filets (6 oz each)
- Salt and pepper to taste
- 2 tablespoons olive oil
- 2 tablespoons fresh lemon juice
- 2 teaspoons dried dill

For Lemon Dill Sauce:

- 1/2 cup Greek yogurt
- 2 tablespoons fresh lemon juice
- 1 tablespoon fresh dill, chopped
- Salt and pepper to taste

For Quinoa Pilaf:

- 1 cup quinoa, rinsed
- 2 cups vegetable broth
- 1 tablespoon olive oil
- 1 small onion, finely chopped
- 2 cloves garlic, minced
- 1/4 cup chopped carrots
- 1/4 cup chopped bell pepper (red or yellow)
- Salt and pepper to taste

For Steamed Broccoli:

- 4 cups broccoli florets

Instructions:

1. Preheat the oven to 400°F (200°C).

2. Season the cod filets with salt and pepper and place them in a baking dish.

3. In a small bowl, mix together olive oil, fresh lemon juice, and dried dill. Pour this mixture over the cod filets, ensuring they are evenly coated.

4. Bake the cod in the preheated oven for 15-20 minutes or until the fish flakes easily with a fork.

5. While the cod is baking, prepare the Lemon Dill Sauce. In a bowl, combine Greek yogurt, fresh lemon juice, chopped dill, salt, and pepper. Mix well and set aside.

6. For the Quinoa Pilaf, rinse the quinoa under cold water. In a saucepan, heat olive oil over medium heat. Add chopped onions and garlic, sauté until softened.

7. Add the rinsed quinoa to the saucepan and stir to coat in the oil. Pour in the vegetable broth, add chopped carrots and bell pepper.

8. Season with salt and pepper. Bring to a boil, then reduce heat, cover, and simmer for 15 minutes or until quinoa is cooked.

9. Steam the broccoli florets until they are tender-crisp, about 5-7 minutes.

10. Once the cod is baked, serve it over a bed of quinoa pilaf, drizzle with Lemon Dill Sauce, and accompany it with steamed broccoli.

11. Garnish with additional fresh dill and lemon slices if desired.

Snack: Almond Butter and Banana Slices on Rice Cakes

Ingredients:

- 4 rice cakes
- 1/2 cup almond butter
- 2 ripe bananas, sliced
- 1 tablespoon honey (optional)
- Chia seeds or sliced almonds for garnish (optional)

Instructions:

1. Spread an even layer of almond butter onto each rice cake.

2. Arrange banana slices on top of the almond butter-covered rice cakes.

3. Drizzle honey over the banana slices for added sweetness if desired.

4. Optionally, sprinkle chia seeds or sliced almonds on top for extra texture and nutrition.

5. Serve the almond butter and banana rice cakes immediately and enjoy a delicious and satisfying snack.

Day 3:

Breakfast: Greek Yogurt Parfait (Greek yogurt, granola, mixed berries, cinnamon)

Ingredients:

- 2 cups Greek yogurt
- 1 cup granola
- 1 cup mixed berries (strawberries, blueberries, raspberries)
- 1/2 teaspoon ground cinnamon
- Honey for drizzling (optional)

Instructions:

1. In serving glasses or bowls, start by layering a spoonful of Greek yogurt at the bottom.

2. Add a layer of granola on top of the Greek yogurt, spreading it evenly.

3. Scatter a handful of mixed berries over the granola layer.

4. Sprinkle a pinch of ground cinnamon over the berries.

5. Repeat the layers until you reach the top of the glass or bowl, finishing with a final layer of mixed berries on top.

6. Optionally, drizzle honey over the parfait for additional sweetness.

7. Serve the Greek Yogurt Parfait immediately and enjoy a delightful and nutritious treat.

Lunch: Mushroom and Barley Soup with a Side Salad

Ingredients:

For Mushroom and Barley Soup:

- 1 cup pearl barley, rinsed
- 8 cups vegetable or mushroom broth
- 2 tablespoons olive oil

- 1 onion, finely chopped
- 3 cloves garlic, minced
- 1 pound (about 500g) mushrooms, sliced (variety of your choice)
- 2 carrots, diced
- 2 celery stalks, chopped
- 1 teaspoon dried thyme
- Salt and pepper to taste
- Fresh parsley for garnish

For Side Salad:

- 4 cups mixed salad greens (lettuce, spinach, arugula, etc.)
- 1 cucumber, sliced
- 1 cup cherry tomatoes, halved
- Balsamic vinaigrette dressing

Instructions:

For Mushroom and Barley Soup:

1. In a large pot, heat olive oil over medium heat. Add chopped onions and garlic, sauté until softened.
2. Add sliced mushrooms to the pot and cook until they release their moisture and become golden brown.

3. Stir in diced carrots and chopped celery. Cook for an additional 5 minutes.

4. Pour in the vegetable or mushroom broth and add the rinsed pearl barley. Season with dried thyme, salt, and pepper.

5. Bring the soup to a boil, then reduce the heat to low, cover, and simmer for about 45-50 minutes or until the barley is tender.

6. Taste the soup and adjust the seasoning if needed. If the soup is too thick, you can add more broth to reach your desired consistency.

7. Garnish the mushroom and barley soup with fresh parsley just before serving.

For Side Salad:

1. In a large bowl, combine mixed salad greens, sliced cucumber, and halved cherry tomatoes.

2. Drizzle balsamic vinaigrette dressing over the salad and toss gently to coat the greens evenly.

3. Serve the Mushroom and Barley Soup with a generous portion of the side salad.

Dinner: Turkey and Vegetable Stir-Fry with Brown Rice

Ingredients:

For the Stir-Fry:

- 1 pound ground turkey
- 2 tablespoons soy sauce
- 1 tablespoon hoisin sauce
- 1 tablespoon oyster sauce
- 1 tablespoon sesame oil
- 1 tablespoon vegetable oil
- 3 cloves garlic, minced
- 1 tablespoon fresh ginger, grated
- 1 cup broccoli florets
- 1 bell pepper, thinly sliced
- 1 carrot, julienned
- 1 cup snap peas, trimmed
- 1 cup cabbage, thinly sliced
- 2 green onions, sliced

For Brown Rice:

- 2 cups brown rice
- 4 cups water
- 1/2 teaspoon salt

Instructions:

For Brown Rice:

1. Rinse the brown rice under cold water.
2. In a medium saucepan, combine the rinsed brown rice, water, and salt. Bring to a boil.
3. Reduce heat to low, cover, and simmer for about 40-45 minutes or until rice is tender and water is absorbed.
4. Once cooked, fluff the rice with a fork.

For Turkey and Vegetable Stir-Fry:

1. In a small bowl, mix together soy sauce, hoisin sauce, and oyster sauce. Set aside.
2. In a large wok or skillet, heat vegetable oil and sesame oil over medium-high heat.
3. Add minced garlic and grated ginger to the hot oil, stirring quickly to release their flavors.
4. Add ground turkey to the wok and cook until browned, breaking it apart with a spatula.
5. Stir in the prepared sauce mixture, ensuring the turkey is well-coated.
6. Add broccoli, bell pepper, julienned carrot, snap peas, and sliced cabbage to the wok. Stir-fry for 5-7 minutes or until the vegetables are tender-crisp.

7. Adjust the seasoning with additional soy sauce or salt if needed.

8. Add sliced green onions and toss for an additional minute.

9. Serve the turkey and vegetable stir-fry over a bed of cooked brown rice.

10. Garnish with additional green onions or sesame seeds if desired.

Snack: Hummus and Veggie Sticks

Ingredients:

For Hummus:

- 1 can (15 oz) chickpeas, drained and rinsed
- 1/4 cup tahini
- 2 cloves garlic, minced
- 3 tablespoons lemon juice
- 2 tablespoons olive oil
- 1/2 teaspoon ground cumin
- Salt and pepper to taste
- 2-3 tablespoons water (as needed for desired consistency)

For Veggie Sticks:

- Carrot sticks
- Cucumber sticks

- Bell pepper strips (assorted colors)
- Celery sticks

Instructions:

For Hummus:

1. In a food processor, combine chickpeas, tahini, minced garlic, lemon juice, olive oil, ground cumin, salt, and pepper.
2. Blend the ingredients until smooth. If the hummus is too thick, add water, one tablespoon at a time, until you reach your desired consistency.
3. Taste and adjust the seasoning as needed.
4. Transfer the hummus to a serving bowl.

For Veggie Sticks:

1. Wash and peel (if desired) the carrots and cucumber. Cut them into sticks.
2. Wash and slice bell peppers into strips.
3. Wash and cut celery into sticks.
4. Arrange the veggie sticks on a serving platter.

To Serve:

1. Place the bowl of hummus in the center of the veggie sticks.

2. Optionally, drizzle a little extra olive oil over the hummus and sprinkle with a pinch of paprika or chopped fresh parsley for garnish.

3. Serve the hummus and veggie sticks as a delicious and healthy appetizer or snack.

Day 4:

Breakfast: Oatmeal with Nut Butter, Sliced Banana, and Flaxseeds

Ingredients:

- 1 cup rolled oats
- 2 cups water or milk (dairy or plant-based)
- Pinch of salt
- 2 tablespoons nut butter (almond, peanut, or your choice)
- 1 ripe banana, sliced
- 1 tablespoon ground flaxseeds
- Optional toppings: honey or maple syrup for sweetness, chopped nuts, or a sprinkle of cinnamon

Instructions:

1. In a saucepan, bring water or milk to a boil.

2. Add rolled oats and a pinch of salt to the boiling liquid. Reduce heat to medium-low and simmer, stirring occasionally, until the oats are tender and the mixture thickens, about 5-7 minutes.

3. Once the oats are cooked, remove the saucepan from heat.

4. Stir in nut butter of your choice until well combined.

5. Transfer the oatmeal to serving bowls.

6. Top the oatmeal with sliced bananas and sprinkle ground flaxseeds on top.

7. If desired, drizzle honey or maple syrup over the oatmeal for added sweetness.

8. Optionally, garnish with chopped nuts or a sprinkle of cinnamon.

9. Serve the oatmeal warm and enjoy a nutritious and filling breakfast.

Lunch: Quinoa Salad with Pomegranate Seeds, Walnuts, and Citrus Dressing

Ingredients:

For the Quinoa Salad:

- 1 cup quinoa, rinsed
- 2 cups water or vegetable broth
- 1 cup pomegranate seeds
- 1/2 cup walnuts, chopped
- 1/2 cup fresh parsley, chopped
- 1/4 cup red onion, finely diced
- 1 cucumber, diced
- 1/2 cup crumbled feta cheese (optional)
- Salt and pepper to taste

For the Citrus Dressing:

- 1/4 cup extra-virgin olive oil
- 2 tablespoons fresh lemon juice
- 1 tablespoon orange juice
- 1 teaspoon honey or maple syrup
- 1 teaspoon Dijon mustard
- Salt and pepper to taste

Instructions:

For Quinoa Salad:

1. In a medium saucepan, combine quinoa and water or vegetable broth. Bring to a boil, then reduce heat to low, cover, and simmer for 15 minutes or until quinoa is cooked and water is absorbed.
2. Once cooked, fluff the quinoa with a fork and allow it to cool to room temperature.
3. In a large salad bowl, combine the cooked quinoa, pomegranate seeds, chopped walnuts, fresh parsley, red onion, cucumber, and crumbled feta cheese (if using).
4. Season the salad with salt and pepper to taste.

For Citrus Dressing:

1. In a small bowl, whisk together extra-virgin olive oil, fresh lemon juice, orange juice, honey or maple syrup, Dijon mustard, salt, and pepper until well combined.
2. Taste the dressing and adjust the sweetness or acidity according to your preference.
3. Pour the citrus dressing over the quinoa salad and toss gently to coat the ingredients evenly.

4. Allow the salad to sit for a few minutes to let the flavors meld.

5. Serve the quinoa salad with pomegranate seeds, walnuts, and citrus dressing chilled or at room temperature.

Dinner: Roasted Butternut Squash Soup, Mixed Green Salad

Ingredients:

For Roasted Butternut Squash Soup:

- 1 large butternut squash, peeled, seeded, and diced
- 1 onion, chopped
- 2 carrots, peeled and chopped
- 3 cloves garlic, minced
- 2 tablespoons olive oil
- 4 cups vegetable broth
- 1 teaspoon ground cumin
- 1/2 teaspoon ground cinnamon
- Salt and pepper to taste
- 1 cup coconut milk (optional, for creaminess)
- Fresh parsley or chives for garnish

For Mixed Green Salad:

- 6 cups mixed salad greens (lettuce, spinach, arugula, etc.)
- 1 cup cherry tomatoes, halved
- 1 cucumber, sliced
- 1/4 red onion, thinly sliced
- Balsamic vinaigrette dressing

Instructions:

For Roasted Butternut Squash Soup:

1. Preheat the oven to 400°F (200°C).
2. In a large mixing bowl, toss the diced butternut squash, chopped onion, carrots, and minced garlic with olive oil, ground cumin, ground cinnamon, salt, and pepper.
3. Spread the seasoned vegetables on a baking sheet in a single layer.
4. Roast in the preheated oven for about 30-35 minutes or until the vegetables are tender and slightly caramelized.
5. Transfer the roasted vegetables to a blender or food processor. Add vegetable broth and blend until smooth.

6. Pour the blended mixture into a large pot. Heat over medium heat, and if desired, add coconut milk for extra creaminess. Stir well.

7. Adjust the seasoning with salt and pepper as needed.

8. Serve the roasted butternut squash soup hot, garnished with fresh parsley or chives.

For Mixed Green Salad:

1. In a large salad bowl, combine mixed salad greens, halved cherry tomatoes, sliced cucumber, and thinly sliced red onion.

2. Drizzle balsamic vinaigrette dressing over the salad and toss gently to coat the greens evenly.

3. Serve the mixed green salad alongside the roasted butternut squash soup.

Snack: Mixed Nuts and Dried Fruits

Ingredients:

- 1 cup almonds
- 1 cup walnuts
- 1 cup cashews
- 1 cup pistachios
- 1 cup mixed dried fruits (apricots, figs, dates, raisins, cranberries, etc.)

- 1 tablespoon olive oil
- 1 teaspoon sea salt (optional)
- 1 teaspoon ground cinnamon (optional)
- 1 tablespoon honey or maple syrup (optional)

Instructions:

1. Preheat the oven to 350°F (175°C).
2. In a large mixing bowl, combine almonds, walnuts, cashews, and pistachios.
3. Toss the nuts with olive oil until they are evenly coated. If desired, add sea salt and ground cinnamon for extra flavor.
4. Spread the coated nuts on a baking sheet in a single layer.
5. Roast the nuts in the preheated oven for 10-15 minutes or until they are golden brown and fragrant. Be sure to stir the nuts occasionally for even roasting.
6. While the nuts are roasting, chop the dried fruits into bite-sized pieces.
7. Once the nuts are roasted, remove them from the oven and let them cool.
8. In a large mixing bowl, combine the roasted nuts with the mixed dried fruits.

9. Optionally, drizzle honey or maple syrup over the mixture and toss until everything is well combined.

10. Allow the mixed nuts and dried fruits to cool completely before transferring them to an airtight container for storage.

Day 5:

Breakfast: Spinach and Feta Omelette with Cherry Tomatoes

Ingredients:

- 3 large eggs
- 1 cup fresh spinach, chopped
- 1/4 cup feta cheese, crumbled
- 1/2 cup cherry tomatoes, halved
- 1 tablespoon olive oil
- Salt and pepper to taste
- Fresh herbs (parsley or chives) for garnish (optional)

Instructions:

1. In a bowl, whisk the eggs until well combined. Season with salt and pepper to taste.

2. Heat olive oil in a non-stick skillet over medium heat.

3. Add chopped fresh spinach to the skillet and sauté for 1-2 minutes until wilted.

4. Pour the whisked eggs over the spinach, ensuring an even distribution.

5. Allow the eggs to set slightly at the edges. As the eggs set, gently lift the edges with a spatula to let the uncooked eggs flow underneath.

6. Once the edges are set and the center is slightly runny, sprinkle crumbled feta cheese evenly over one half of the omelette.

7. Add halved cherry tomatoes on top of the feta cheese.

8. Carefully fold the other half of the omelette over the filling, creating a half-moon shape.

9. Cook for an additional 1-2 minutes until the cheese starts to melt, and the tomatoes are heated through.

10. Slide the omelette onto a plate, garnish with fresh herbs if desired, and serve immediately.

Lunch: Vegetable and Quinoa Stuffed Bell Peppers

Ingredients:

- 4 large bell peppers, halved and seeds removed
- 1 cup quinoa, rinsed
- 2 cups vegetable broth
- 2 tablespoons olive oil
- 1 onion, finely chopped
- 2 cloves garlic, minced
- 1 carrot, diced
- 1 zucchini, diced
- 1 cup cherry tomatoes, halved
- 1 cup corn kernels (fresh, frozen, or canned)
- 1 teaspoon dried oregano
- 1 teaspoon ground cumin
- Salt and pepper to taste
- 1 cup shredded cheese (cheddar, mozzarella, or your choice)
- Fresh parsley or cilantro for garnish (optional)

Instructions:

1. Preheat the oven to 375°F (190°C).
2. In a medium saucepan, combine quinoa and vegetable broth.

3. Bring to a boil, then reduce heat to low, cover, and simmer for 15 minutes or until quinoa is cooked and liquid is absorbed.
4. While the quinoa is cooking, heat olive oil in a large skillet over medium heat.
5. Add chopped onion and minced garlic to the skillet. Sauté until the onion is softened.
6. Add diced carrot and zucchini to the skillet and cook for an additional 5 minutes until the vegetables are tender.
7. Stir in halved cherry tomatoes and corn kernels. Season with dried oregano, ground cumin, salt, and pepper. Cook for another 2-3 minutes.
8. Once the quinoa is cooked, fluff it with a fork and add it to the vegetable mixture. Mix well to combine.
9. Arrange the bell pepper halves in a baking dish.
10. Spoon the quinoa and vegetable mixture into each bell pepper half.
11. Top each stuffed pepper with shredded cheese.
12. Cover the baking dish with foil and bake in the preheated oven for 25-30 minutes or until the peppers are tender.

13. If desired, broil for an additional 2-3 minutes to melt and brown the cheese.

14. Garnish with fresh parsley or cilantro before serving.

Dinner: Grilled Turkey Burger with Sweet Potato Fries, Side Salad

Ingredients:

For Grilled Turkey Burger:

- 1 pound ground turkey
- 1/4 cup breadcrumbs
- 1 egg
- 1/4 cup grated Parmesan cheese
- 2 cloves garlic, minced
- 1 teaspoon dried oregano
- Salt and pepper to taste
- 4 whole-grain burger buns
- Lettuce, tomato slices, and red onion for garnish

For Sweet Potato Fries:

- 2 large sweet potatoes, peeled and cut into fries
- 2 tablespoons olive oil
- 1 teaspoon paprika
- 1/2 teaspoon garlic powder
- Salt and pepper to taste

For Side Salad:

- 6 cups mixed salad greens (lettuce, spinach, arugula, etc.)
- 1 cup cherry tomatoes, halved
- 1 cucumber, sliced
- Balsamic vinaigrette dressing

Instructions:

For Grilled Turkey Burger:

1. In a bowl, combine ground turkey, breadcrumbs, egg, grated Parmesan cheese, minced garlic, dried oregano, salt, and pepper.
2. Mix the ingredients until well combined, and then shape the mixture into four burger patties.
3. Preheat the grill to medium-high heat.
4. Grill the turkey burgers for approximately 5-6 minutes per side or until fully cooked and internal temperature reaches 165°F (74°C).
5. Toast the whole-grain burger buns on the grill during the last 1-2 minutes of cooking.
6. Assemble the burgers with lettuce, tomato slices, and red onion on the toasted buns.

For Sweet Potato Fries:

1. Preheat the oven to 425°F (220°C).

2. In a large bowl, toss sweet potato fries with olive oil, paprika, garlic powder, salt, and pepper until evenly coated.

3. Spread the sweet potato fries in a single layer on a baking sheet.

4. Bake in the preheated oven for 25-30 minutes or until the fries are golden and crispy, flipping them halfway through.

For Side Salad:

1. In a large salad bowl, combine mixed salad greens, halved cherry tomatoes, and sliced cucumber.

2. Drizzle balsamic vinaigrette dressing over the salad and toss gently to coat the greens evenly.

3. Serve the side salad alongside the grilled turkey burger and sweet potato fries.

Snack: Cottage Cheese with Pineapple

Ingredients:

- 1 cup cottage cheese
- 1 cup fresh pineapple chunks (or canned pineapple tidbits, drained)
- 1 tablespoon honey (optional)

- 2 tablespoons chopped nuts (walnuts, almonds, or your choice)
- Mint leaves for garnish (optional)

Instructions:

1. Spoon the cottage cheese into a serving bowl.
2. Add fresh pineapple chunks on top of the cottage cheese.
3. If desired, drizzle honey over the cottage cheese and pineapple for added sweetness.
4. Sprinkle chopped nuts over the mixture for extra crunch and flavor.
5. Garnish with mint leaves for a fresh touch (optional).
6. Serve the cottage cheese with pineapple immediately and enjoy a simple and nutritious snack or breakfast.

Day 6:

Breakfast: Smoothie Bowl (spinach, banana, berries, almond milk, topped with kiwi and chia seeds)

Ingredients:

For the Smoothie Base:

- 1 cup fresh spinach leaves
- 1 frozen banana, sliced
- 1/2 cup mixed berries (strawberries, blueberries, raspberries)
- 1 cup almond milk (or any milk of your choice)
- 1 tablespoon chia seeds

Toppings:

- 1 kiwi, peeled and sliced
- 1 tablespoon chia seeds

Optional Garnish:

- Granola
- Shredded coconut
- Sliced almonds

Instructions:

1. In a blender, combine fresh spinach leaves, frozen banana slices, mixed berries, almond milk, and chia seeds.
2. Blend the ingredients until smooth and creamy. If needed, add more almond milk to achieve your desired consistency.
3. Pour the smoothie into a bowl.
4. Arrange sliced kiwi on top of the smoothie bowl.
5. Sprinkle chia seeds over the smoothie.
6. Optionally, garnish with additional toppings like granola, shredded coconut, or sliced almonds.
7. Serve the smoothie bowl immediately and enjoy a refreshing and nutritious meal.

Lunch: Red Lentil and Sweet Potato Soup with Whole Grain Roll

Ingredients:

For Red Lentil and Sweet Potato Soup:
- 1 cup red lentils, rinsed
- 1 large sweet potato, peeled and diced
- 1 onion, chopped
- 2 carrots, peeled and sliced
- 3 cloves garlic, minced

- 1 teaspoon ground cumin
- 1 teaspoon ground coriander
- 1/2 teaspoon smoked paprika
- 6 cups vegetable broth
- 1 can (14 oz) diced tomatoes
- Salt and pepper to taste
- 2 tablespoons olive oil
- Fresh cilantro or parsley for garnish

For Whole Grain Roll:

- 4 whole grain rolls

Instructions:

For Red Lentil and Sweet Potato Soup:

1. In a large pot, heat olive oil over medium heat. Add chopped onion and minced garlic. Sauté until the onion is softened.

2. Add ground cumin, ground coriander, and smoked paprika to the pot. Stir well to coat the onions and garlic with the spices.

3. Add diced sweet potato and sliced carrots to the pot. Cook for 5 minutes, stirring occasionally.

4. Pour in vegetable broth, add rinsed red lentils, and bring the mixture to a boil.

5. Reduce the heat to low, cover, and simmer for about 20-25 minutes or until the lentils and vegetables are tender.

6. Add diced tomatoes (with their juice) to the soup. Season with salt and pepper to taste. Simmer for an additional 10 minutes.

7. Taste the soup and adjust the seasoning if needed.

8. Ladle the red lentil and sweet potato soup into bowls, garnish with fresh cilantro or parsley, and serve hot.

For Whole Grain Roll:

1. Preheat the oven according to the instructions on the whole grain roll package.

2. Place the whole grain rolls on a baking sheet.

3. Bake the rolls in the preheated oven until they are golden brown and crusty.

4. Serve the whole grain rolls alongside the red lentil and sweet potato soup.

Dinner: Chickpea and Vegetable Stir-Fry with Quinoa

Ingredients:

For the Stir-Fry:

- 1 cup cooked chickpeas (canned or cooked from dried)
- 1 cup broccoli florets
- 1 bell pepper, thinly sliced
- 1 carrot, julienned
- 1 zucchini, sliced
- 2 cups snow peas, ends trimmed
- 3 tablespoons soy sauce
- 2 tablespoons sesame oil
- 1 tablespoon hoisin sauce
- 1 tablespoon rice vinegar
- 1 tablespoon grated ginger
- 2 cloves garlic, minced
- 1 tablespoon olive oil
- 4 cups cooked quinoa

Instructions:

1. In a small bowl, mix together soy sauce, sesame oil, hoisin sauce, and rice vinegar. Set aside.
2. Heat olive oil in a large wok or skillet over medium-high heat.

3. Add minced garlic and grated ginger to the hot oil, stirring quickly to release their flavors.

4. Add sliced bell pepper, julienned carrot, sliced zucchini, broccoli florets, and snow peas to the wok. Stir-fry for 5-7 minutes or until the vegetables are tender-crisp.

5. Add cooked chickpeas to the wok and pour the sauce mixture over the vegetables and chickpeas. Toss everything together to ensure an even coating.

6. Continue to stir-fry for an additional 2-3 minutes until the chickpeas are heated through and the sauce has coated the vegetables.

7. In a separate pan or using the same wok, stir-fry the cooked quinoa for 2-3 minutes until it's heated through.

8. Serve the chickpea and vegetable stir-fry over a bed of cooked quinoa.

Snack: Apple Slices with Nut Butter

Ingredients:

- 2 apples (your choice of variety), cored and sliced

- 1/2 cup nut butter (almond, peanut, or your choice)
- 2 tablespoons honey or maple syrup (optional)
- 2 tablespoons chopped nuts (walnuts, almonds, or pecans)
- 1 teaspoon ground cinnamon (optional)

Instructions:

1. Core and slice the apples into wedges or rings.
2. In a small microwave-safe bowl, warm the nut butter for about 20-30 seconds until it becomes smooth and slightly runny.
3. Arrange the apple slices on a serving plate.
4. Drizzle the warmed nut butter over the apple slices. If desired, also drizzle honey or maple syrup for added sweetness.
5. Sprinkle chopped nuts over the nut butter-covered apple slices.
6. Optionally, dust the apple slices with ground cinnamon for extra flavor.
7. Serve the apple slices with nut butter immediately and enjoy as a healthy snack or dessert.

Day 7:

Breakfast: Whole Grain Pancakes with Mixed Berries and Maple Syrup

Ingredients:

For Whole Grain Pancakes:

- 1 cup whole wheat flour
- 1/2 cup oat flour
- 2 tablespoons ground flaxseed
- 1 tablespoon baking powder
- 1/2 teaspoon baking soda
- 1/4 teaspoon salt
- 1 cup buttermilk (or milk of your choice)
- 1 large egg
- 2 tablespoons melted butter or oil
- 1 tablespoon honey or maple syrup
- 1 teaspoon vanilla extract

For Toppings:

- Mixed berries (strawberries, blueberries, raspberries)
- Maple syrup
- Additional melted butter (optional)

Instructions:

1. In a large mixing bowl, whisk together whole wheat flour, oat flour, ground flaxseed, baking powder, baking soda, and salt.

2. In a separate bowl, whisk together buttermilk, egg, melted butter or oil, honey or maple syrup, and vanilla extract.

3. Pour the wet ingredients into the dry ingredients and stir until just combined. Be careful not to overmix; some lumps are okay.

4. Let the batter rest for a few minutes while you preheat a griddle or non-stick skillet over medium heat.

5. Lightly grease the griddle or skillet with butter or oil.

6. Pour 1/4 cup portions of batter onto the hot griddle to form pancakes. Cook until bubbles form on the surface, then flip and cook the other side until golden brown.

7. Repeat until all the batter is used, keeping cooked pancakes warm in a low oven if needed.

8. Meanwhile, wash and prepare the mixed berries.

9. Stack the whole grain pancakes on serving plates.

10. Top with mixed berries and drizzle with maple syrup. Optionally, add a pat of melted butter.

11. Serve the whole grain pancakes with mixed berries and maple syrup immediately, and enjoy a wholesome and delicious breakfast.

Lunch: Fish and Vegetable Chowder with a Side of Quinoa

Ingredients:

For Fish and Vegetable Chowder:

- 1 pound white fish filets (cod, haddock, or your choice), cut into chunks
- 1 onion, finely chopped
- 2 carrots, diced
- 2 celery stalks, sliced
- 2 potatoes, peeled and diced
- 2 cloves garlic, minced
- 4 cups fish or vegetable broth
- 1 cup corn kernels (fresh, frozen, or canned)
- 1 cup green beans, trimmed and cut into bite-sized pieces
- 1 cup milk or cream
- 2 tablespoons all-purpose flour
- 2 tablespoons butter

- 1 bay leaf
- Salt and pepper to taste
- Fresh parsley for garnish

For Quinoa:

- 1 cup quinoa, rinsed
- 2 cups water
- 1/2 teaspoon salt

Instructions:

For Fish and Vegetable Chowder:

1. In a large pot, melt butter over medium heat. Add chopped onion and garlic, sautéing until softened.

2. Add diced carrots, celery, and potatoes to the pot. Cook for 5 minutes, stirring occasionally.

3. Sprinkle flour over the vegetables, stirring to coat them evenly. Cook for an additional 2 minutes to remove the raw taste of the flour.

4. Gradually add fish or vegetable broth to the pot, stirring constantly to avoid lumps.

5. Add bay leaf, salt, and pepper to taste. Bring the mixture to a simmer, then reduce heat and let it simmer until the vegetables are tender.

6. Stir in fish chunks, corn kernels, and green beans. Simmer for an additional 5-7 minutes or until the fish is cooked through.

7. Pour in milk or cream, stirring gently to combine. Simmer for an additional 2-3 minutes.

8. Taste and adjust the seasoning if necessary. Remove the bay leaf.

9. Garnish the fish and vegetable chowder with fresh parsley before serving.

For Quinoa:

1. Rinse quinoa under cold water.

2. In a saucepan, combine rinsed quinoa, water, and salt. Bring to a boil.

3. Reduce heat to low, cover, and simmer for about 15 minutes or until quinoa is cooked and water is absorbed.

4. Fluff the quinoa with a fork.

To Serve:

1. Spoon the fish and vegetable chowder into bowls.

2. Serve with a side of cooked quinoa.

Dinner: Stuffed Acorn Squash with Turkey, Quinoa, and Cranberries

Ingredients:

- 2 acorn squashes, halved and seeds removed
- 1 cup quinoa, rinsed
- 2 cups chicken or vegetable broth
- 1 tablespoon olive oil
- 1 onion, finely chopped
- 1 pound ground turkey
- 2 cloves garlic, minced
- 1 teaspoon ground cumin
- 1 teaspoon ground cinnamon
- 1/2 teaspoon ground nutmeg
- Salt and pepper to taste
- 1/2 cup dried cranberries
- 1/2 cup chopped pecans or walnuts
- 1/4 cup chopped fresh parsley
- 1/4 cup feta cheese, crumbled (optional)
- 2 tablespoons maple syrup (optional, for drizzling)

Instructions:

1. Preheat the oven to 400°F (200°C).
2. Place the acorn squash halves on a baking sheet, cut side up.

3. Drizzle with olive oil and sprinkle with salt and pepper. Roast in the preheated oven for 30-35 minutes or until the squash is tender.

4. While the squash is roasting, prepare the quinoa. In a saucepan, combine quinoa and broth. Bring to a boil, then reduce heat to low, cover, and simmer for 15 minutes or until quinoa is cooked and liquid is absorbed.

5. In a large skillet, heat olive oil over medium heat. Add chopped onion and sauté until softened.

6. Add ground turkey to the skillet, breaking it apart with a spoon. Cook until browned.

7. Add minced garlic, ground cumin, ground cinnamon, ground nutmeg, salt, and pepper to the skillet. Stir well to combine.

8. Once the turkey is cooked through and the spices are fragrant, add cooked quinoa, dried cranberries, chopped nuts, and fresh parsley to the skillet. Mix until well combined.

9. Adjust seasoning if needed. Optionally, stir in crumbled feta cheese.

10. Remove the acorn squash halves from the oven. Fill each squash half with the turkey and quinoa mixture.

11. Drizzle maple syrup over the stuffed squash if desired.

12. Return the stuffed acorn squash to the oven and bake for an additional 10-15 minutes or until heated through.

13. Serve the stuffed acorn squash with turkey, quinoa, and cranberries hot from the oven.

Snack: Roasted Chickpeas

Ingredients:

- 2 cans (15 oz each) chickpeas (garbanzo beans), drained and rinsed
- 2 tablespoons olive oil
- 1 teaspoon ground cumin
- 1 teaspoon smoked paprika
- 1/2 teaspoon garlic powder
- 1/2 teaspoon onion powder
- 1/4 teaspoon cayenne pepper (adjust to taste for spiciness)
- Salt to taste

Instructions:

1. Preheat the oven to 400°F (200°C).
2. Rinse and drain the chickpeas. Pat them dry with a clean kitchen towel to remove excess moisture.
3. In a large bowl, combine the chickpeas with olive oil, ground cumin, smoked paprika, garlic powder, onion powder, cayenne pepper, and salt. Toss until the chickpeas are evenly coated with the spices.
4. Spread the chickpeas in a single layer on a baking sheet lined with parchment paper.
5. Roast in the preheated oven for 25-30 minutes, shaking the pan halfway through to ensure even roasting. The chickpeas should be golden brown and crispy.
6. Once roasted, remove the chickpeas from the oven and let them cool for a few minutes.
7. Taste and adjust the seasoning if needed. Add a bit more salt or spice according to your preference.
8. Serve the roasted chickpeas as a snack on their own or use them as a crunchy topping for salads, soups, or yogurt.

"I nourish my body with wholesome foods, supporting my journey to recovery."

"My positive thoughts contribute to the healing energy within me."

CHAPTER 3: BREAKFAST

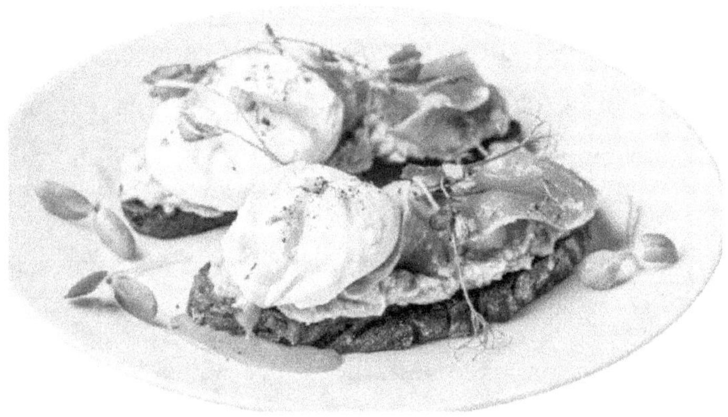

Quinoa Breakfast Bowl

Ingredients:

- 1 cup quinoa
- 2 cups almond milk (or any milk of your choice)
- 1 tablespoon honey or maple syrup
- 1 teaspoon vanilla extract
- 1/2 teaspoon cinnamon
- Pinch of salt
- Fresh fruits (berries, banana slices, etc.)
- Nuts and seeds (almonds, chia seeds, etc.)
- Greek yogurt or coconut yogurt
- Optional toppings: shredded coconut, granola, or additional honey

1. Rinse the quinoa under cold water to remove any bitterness.

2. In a saucepan, combine the quinoa, almond milk, honey or maple syrup, vanilla extract, cinnamon, and a pinch of salt. Bring to a boil, then reduce the heat to low, cover, and simmer for about 15-20 minutes or until the quinoa is cooked and the liquid is absorbed.

3. Once cooked, fluff the quinoa with a fork and let it cool for a few minutes.

4. In serving bowls, spoon the cooked quinoa.

5. Top the quinoa with fresh fruits, nuts, seeds, and a dollop of Greek yogurt or coconut yogurt.

6. Add any optional toppings like shredded coconut, granola, or an extra drizzle of honey for sweetness.

7. Mix everything together before enjoying your nutritious and flavorful quinoa breakfast bowl!

Avocado Toast with Salmon

Ingredients:

- 2 slices of whole-grain bread
- 1 ripe avocado

- 1 tablespoon lemon juice
- Salt and pepper to taste
- 100g smoked salmon
- 1 tablespoon capers
- Fresh dill for garnish
- Optional: poached or fried egg for extra protein

Instructions:

1. Toast the slices of whole-grain bread to your liking.
2. While the bread is toasting, cut the ripe avocado in half, remove the pit, and scoop the flesh into a bowl. Mash the avocado with a fork.
3. Add lemon juice, salt, and pepper to the mashed avocado. Mix well until you have a creamy avocado spread.
4. Once the bread is toasted, spread the mashed avocado evenly over each slice.
5. Layer smoked salmon over the avocado on each slice of toast.
6. Sprinkle capers over the salmon. Capers add a briny flavor that complements the richness of the salmon.
7. Garnish with fresh dill for added freshness and flavor.

8. If desired, top each toast with a poached or fried egg for extra protein and richness.

9. Season with additional salt and pepper to taste.

10. Serve immediately and enjoy your delicious and nutritious Avocado Toast with Salmon!

Greek Yogurt Parfait

Ingredients:

- 1 cup Greek yogurt (plain or flavored)
- 1/2 cup granola
- 1/2 cup mixed berries (strawberries, blueberries, raspberries)
- 1 tablespoon honey
- 1/4 cup chopped nuts (almonds, walnuts, or your choice)
- Optional: a sprinkle of cinnamon for added flavor

Instructions:

1. In a serving glass or bowl, start by spooning a layer of Greek yogurt at the bottom.

2. Add a layer of granola on top of the Greek yogurt. This provides a nice crunch and additional texture.

3. Wash and prepare the mixed berries. Place a layer of berries over the granola.

4. Drizzle a tablespoon of honey over the berries. Adjust the amount based on your sweetness preference.

5. Sprinkle a layer of chopped nuts over the honey. This adds a delightful nutty flavor and extra crunch.

6. Repeat the layers until you fill the glass or bowl, ending with a topping of berries and a drizzle of honey.

7. Optional: Sprinkle a pinch of cinnamon over the top for added warmth and flavor.

8. Serve immediately and enjoy your delicious and nutritious Greek Yogurt Parfait!

Oatmeal with Nut Butter

Ingredients:

- 1/2 cup old-fashioned rolled oats
- 1 cup milk (dairy or plant-based)
- 1 tablespoon nut butter (peanut butter, almond butter, or your choice)
- 1 tablespoon honey or maple syrup
- 1/2 teaspoon vanilla extract

- Pinch of salt
- Toppings: sliced banana, chopped nuts, and a sprinkle of cinnamon

Instructions:

1. In a saucepan, combine the rolled oats and milk. Bring to a gentle boil over medium heat, then reduce the heat to low and simmer, stirring occasionally, until the oats are soft and the mixture has thickened (usually about 5-7 minutes).

2. Once the oats are cooked, stir in the nut butter of your choice. The heat from the oatmeal will help melt the nut butter and create a creamy consistency.

3. Add honey or maple syrup, vanilla extract, and a pinch of salt. Stir well to combine.

4. Remove the oatmeal from the heat and let it sit for a minute to allow it to thicken further.

5. Spoon the oatmeal into a bowl and top it with sliced bananas, chopped nuts, and a sprinkle of cinnamon.

6. Optionally, drizzle a little extra honey or add a dollop of yogurt on top for additional sweetness and creaminess.

7. Serve warm and enjoy your comforting bowl of Oatmeal with Nut Butter!

Egg and Vegetable Scramble

Ingredients:

- 2 large eggs
- 1 tablespoon olive oil or butter
- 1/4 cup diced onion
- 1/2 cup diced bell peppers (any color)
- 1/2 cup diced tomatoes
- 1/4 cup diced mushrooms
- Salt and pepper to taste
- Optional: shredded cheese, chopped fresh herbs (parsley, chives), hot sauce

Instructions:

1. Heat olive oil or butter in a skillet over medium heat.
2. Add diced onions to the skillet and sauté until they become translucent.
3. Add diced bell peppers to the skillet and cook for a few minutes until they start to soften.
4. Stir in diced mushrooms and cook until they release their moisture and become tender.

5. Add diced tomatoes to the mixture and cook briefly until they are heated through but still retain their shape.

6. In a bowl, whisk the eggs together and season with salt and pepper.

7. Push the vegetables to the side of the skillet, pour the whisked eggs into the empty space, and let them sit for a moment.

8. Using a spatula, gently scramble the eggs, incorporating them with the sautéed vegetables.

9. Continue stirring until the eggs are cooked to your desired level of doneness.

10. Optional: Sprinkle shredded cheese over the scramble and let it melt for added richness.

11. Garnish with chopped fresh herbs, and if you like it spicy, add a dash of hot sauce.

12. Serve the Egg and Vegetable Scramble hot, either on its own or with toast or tortillas on the side.

Smoothie Bowl

Ingredients:

- 1 frozen banana, sliced

- 1 cup frozen mixed berries (strawberries, blueberries, raspberries)
- 1/2 cup Greek yogurt
- 1/2 cup almond milk (or any milk of your choice)
- 1 tablespoon honey or maple syrup (optional, for sweetness)
- Toppings: sliced fresh fruits, granola, chia seeds, shredded coconut, nuts, and seeds

Instructions:

1. In a blender, combine the frozen banana slices, frozen mixed berries, Greek yogurt, and almond milk.
2. Blend the ingredients until smooth and creamy. If the mixture is too thick, you can add more almond milk in small increments until you reach your desired consistency.
3. Taste the smoothie and add honey or maple syrup if you prefer a sweeter flavor. Blend again to incorporate.
4. Pour the smoothie into a bowl.

5. Arrange your desired toppings on the smoothie. This could include sliced fresh fruits, granola for crunch, chia seeds for added texture, shredded coconut for sweetness, and a variety of nuts and seeds for extra nutrition.

6. Get creative with the arrangement of toppings, making your smoothie bowl visually appealing.

7. Optionally, drizzle a bit more honey or sprinkle a dash of cinnamon on top for extra flavor.

8. Serve immediately and enjoy your vibrant and nutritious Smoothie Bowl!

Chia Seed Pudding

Ingredients:

- 1/4 cup chia seeds
- 1 cup milk (dairy or plant-based)
- 1 tablespoon honey or maple syrup
- 1/2 teaspoon vanilla extract
- Toppings: sliced fruits, berries, nuts, and a drizzle of honey

Instructions:

1. In a bowl, combine chia seeds, milk, honey or maple syrup, and vanilla extract.

2. Whisk the mixture thoroughly to ensure the chia seeds are well distributed and don't clump together.

3. Let the mixture sit for about 5 minutes, then whisk again to prevent clumps from forming.

4. Cover the bowl and refrigerate for at least 2-3 hours, or preferably overnight. The chia seeds will absorb the liquid and create a pudding-like consistency.

5. After refrigeration, give the pudding a good stir to break up any remaining clumps and ensure a smooth texture.

6. Spoon the chia seed pudding into serving bowls or jars.

7. Top the pudding with sliced fruits, berries, and your favorite nuts.

8. Optionally, drizzle a bit of honey over the top for added sweetness.

9. Serve chilled and enjoy your delicious and nutritious Chia Seed Pudding!

Sweet Potato Hash

Ingredients:

- 2 medium sweet potatoes, peeled and diced

- 1 onion, finely chopped
- 1 bell pepper, diced (any color)
- 2 cloves garlic, minced
- 2 tablespoons olive oil
- 1 teaspoon smoked paprika
- 1/2 teaspoon cumin
- 1/2 teaspoon chili powder (adjust to taste)
- Salt and pepper to taste
- 2 cups spinach or kale, chopped
- Optional toppings: poached or fried eggs, avocado slices, hot sauce

Instructions:

1. In a large skillet, heat olive oil over medium heat.
2. Add chopped onions to the skillet and sauté until they become translucent.
3. Add diced sweet potatoes to the skillet. Cook for about 10-15 minutes or until they are tender and slightly crispy on the edges. Stir occasionally to ensure even cooking.
4. Add diced bell pepper and minced garlic to the sweet potatoes. Cook for an additional 5 minutes until the bell peppers are tender.

5. Sprinkle smoked paprika, cumin, chili powder, salt, and pepper over the sweet potato mixture. Stir well to coat evenly with the spices.

6. Add chopped spinach or kale to the skillet. Stir until the greens are wilted and well combined with the sweet potato mixture.

7. Continue cooking for a few more minutes until everything is heated through and well blended.

8. Adjust seasoning if necessary.

9. Optional: Top the sweet potato hash with poached or fried eggs for extra protein and richness.

10. Serve hot and garnish with avocado slices and a drizzle of hot sauce if desired.

Cottage Cheese and Pineapple Plate

Ingredients:
- 1 cup cottage cheese
- 1 cup fresh pineapple chunks
- 1/4 cup chopped fresh mint (optional, for garnish)
- 2 tablespoons honey or maple syrup
- 1/4 cup chopped nuts (walnuts, almonds, or your choice)

- Optional: a sprinkle of cinnamon for added flavor

Instructions:

1. In a serving plate or bowl, arrange the cottage cheese.
2. Add fresh pineapple chunks on top of the cottage cheese.
3. Drizzle honey or maple syrup over the cottage cheese and pineapple.
4. Sprinkle chopped nuts over the mixture. This adds a delightful crunch and extra protein.
5. Optional: Sprinkle a pinch of cinnamon for added warmth and flavor.
6. Garnish with chopped fresh mint for a burst of freshness.
7. Give everything a gentle toss or leave it layered, depending on your preference.
8. Serve immediately and enjoy your Cottage Cheese and Pineapple Plate!

Brown Rice Porridge

Ingredients:

- 1 cup brown rice
- 4 cups water

- 2 cups milk (dairy or plant-based)
- 2 tablespoons maple syrup or honey
- 1 teaspoon vanilla extract
- 1/2 teaspoon cinnamon
- Pinch of salt
- Toppings: sliced banana, chopped nuts, dried fruits, and a sprinkle of cinnamon

Instructions:

1. Rinse the brown rice under cold water.
2. In a large saucepan, combine the rinsed brown rice and water. Bring it to a boil over high heat.
3. Reduce the heat to low, cover the saucepan, and let it simmer for about 45-50 minutes or until the rice is tender and has absorbed most of the water.
4. Once the rice is cooked, add milk to the saucepan. Stir well and continue simmering over low heat.
5. Add maple syrup or honey, vanilla extract, cinnamon, and a pinch of salt to the rice and milk mixture. Stir to combine.

6. Continue simmering the mixture for an additional 15-20 minutes, or until it reaches your desired porridge consistency. Stir occasionally to prevent sticking.

7. Taste and adjust sweetness if needed.

8. Serve the brown rice porridge warm in bowls.

9. Top with sliced banana, chopped nuts, dried fruits, and a sprinkle of cinnamon.

10. Optionally, drizzle a bit more maple syrup or honey over the top for added sweetness.

11. Enjoy your wholesome and delicious Brown Rice Porridge!

Spinach and Feta Omelette

Ingredients:

- 3 large eggs
- 1 cup fresh spinach, chopped
- 1/4 cup feta cheese, crumbled
- 1/4 cup diced tomatoes
- 1/4 cup diced red bell pepper
- 1/4 cup diced onion
- 1 tablespoon olive oil or butter
- Salt and pepper to taste
- Fresh herbs (optional, for garnish)

Instructions:

1. Crack the eggs into a bowl and beat them with a fork or whisk until well combined. Season with a pinch of salt and pepper.
2. Heat olive oil or butter in a non-stick skillet over medium heat.
3. Add diced onions and sauté until they become translucent.
4. Add diced red bell pepper to the skillet and cook for a few minutes until it starts to soften.
5. Add chopped spinach to the skillet and cook until it wilts, stirring occasionally.
6. Pour the beaten eggs over the sautéed vegetables in the skillet.
7. Allow the eggs to set slightly at the edges, then gently lift the edges with a spatula, tilting the skillet to let the uncooked eggs flow underneath.
8. When the omelette is mostly set but still slightly runny on top, sprinkle crumbled feta cheese and diced tomatoes over one half of the omelette.
9. Carefully fold the other half of the omelette over the filling, creating a half-moon shape.

10. Press down gently with the spatula and let it cook for another minute or until the eggs are cooked through.

11. Slide the omelette onto a plate and garnish with fresh herbs if desired.

12. Serve hot and enjoy your delicious Spinach and Feta Omelette!

Whole Grain Pancakes

Ingredients:

- 1 cup whole wheat flour
- 1/4 cup oats
- 1 tablespoon flaxseed meal
- 1 tablespoon baking powder
- 1/2 teaspoon cinnamon
- 1/4 teaspoon salt
- 1 cup milk (dairy or plant-based)
- 1 large egg
- 2 tablespoons maple syrup or honey
- 2 tablespoons melted butter or oil
- 1 teaspoon vanilla extract

Instructions:

1. In a large mixing bowl, combine whole wheat flour, oats, flaxseed meal, baking powder, cinnamon, and salt.
2. In a separate bowl, whisk together milk, egg, maple syrup or honey, melted butter or oil, and vanilla extract.
3. Pour the wet ingredients into the dry ingredients. Stir until just combined. The batter may be a bit lumpy; avoid overmixing.
4. Let the batter rest for a few minutes to allow the oats to absorb some liquid.
5. Preheat a griddle or non-stick skillet over medium heat. Lightly grease it with cooking spray or a small amount of butter.
6. Pour 1/4 cup of batter onto the griddle for each pancake. Cook until bubbles form on the surface and the edges begin to look set, usually 2-3 minutes.
7. Flip the pancakes and cook for an additional 1-2 minutes, or until golden brown and cooked through.
8. Repeat with the remaining batter, adjusting the heat as needed.

9. Keep the pancakes warm in a low oven until ready to serve.

10. Serve the whole grain pancakes with your favorite toppings such as fresh fruit, a dollop of Greek yogurt, or a drizzle of maple syrup.

11. Enjoy your nutritious and delicious Whole Grain Pancakes!

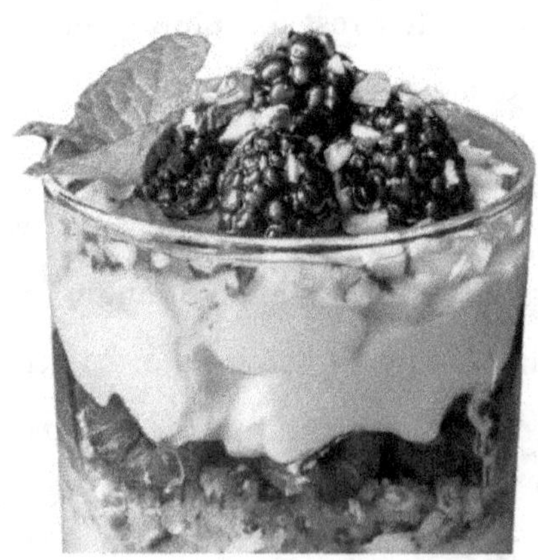

CHAPTER 4: LUNCH

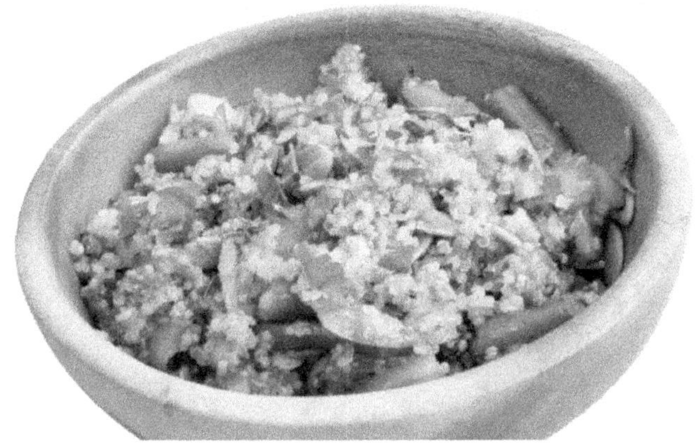

Grilled Chicken Salad

Ingredients:

- 1 pound boneless, skinless chicken breasts
- Salt and pepper to taste
- 2 tablespoons olive oil
- 1 teaspoon dried oregano
- 1 teaspoon garlic powder
- 1 teaspoon paprika
- 1 teaspoon onion powder
- 6 cups mixed salad greens (lettuce, spinach, arugula, etc.)
- 1 cup cherry tomatoes, halved
- 1 cucumber, sliced

- 1 bell pepper, sliced

- 1/2 red onion, thinly sliced

- 1/2 cup Kalamata olives, pitted

- 1/2 cup feta cheese, crumbled

For the dressing:

- 1/4 cup extra virgin olive oil

- 2 tablespoons red wine vinegar

- 1 teaspoon Dijon mustard

- 1 teaspoon honey

- Salt and pepper to taste

Instructions:

1. Preheat the grill to medium-high heat.

2. Season the chicken breasts with salt, pepper, oregano, garlic powder, paprika, and onion powder. Drizzle with olive oil and rub the seasonings into the chicken.

3. Grill the chicken breasts for about 6-8 minutes per side or until the internal temperature reaches 165°F (74°C). Cooking time may vary depending on the thickness of the chicken. Once cooked, let the chicken rest for a few minutes before slicing it into strips.

4. While the chicken is grilling, prepare the salad by combining the mixed greens, cherry tomatoes, cucumber, bell pepper, red onion, Kalamata olives, and feta cheese in a large bowl.

5. In a small bowl, whisk together the dressing ingredients: extra virgin olive oil, red wine vinegar, Dijon mustard, honey, salt, and pepper.

6. Pour the dressing over the salad and toss to coat the ingredients evenly.

7. Once the chicken is sliced, arrange the grilled chicken strips on top of the salad.

8. Serve immediately and enjoy your delicious Grilled Chicken Salad!

Quinoa and Vegetable Stir-Fry

Ingredients:

- 1 cup quinoa, rinsed and drained
- 2 cups water or vegetable broth
- 2 tablespoons vegetable oil
- 1 onion, thinly sliced
- 2 cloves garlic, minced
- 1 red bell pepper, thinly sliced
- 1 yellow bell pepper, thinly sliced
- 1 zucchini, diced

- 1 cup broccoli florets
- 1 carrot, julienned
- 1 cup snap peas, trimmed
- 1/4 cup soy sauce
- 2 tablespoons hoisin sauce
- 1 tablespoon sesame oil
- 1 teaspoon grated fresh ginger
- 2 green onions, chopped (for garnish)
- Sesame seeds (optional, for garnish)

Instructions:

1. In a medium saucepan, combine quinoa and water or vegetable broth. Bring to a boil, then reduce heat to low, cover, and simmer for about 15 minutes or until the quinoa is cooked and water is absorbed. Fluff with a fork and set aside.

2. Heat vegetable oil in a large skillet or wok over medium-high heat.

3. Add sliced onion and minced garlic to the skillet, sautéing for 2-3 minutes until softened and fragrant.

4. Add the sliced red and yellow bell peppers, diced zucchini, broccoli florets, julienned carrot, and snap peas to the skillet.

5. Stir-fry the vegetables for 5-7 minutes or until they are tender-crisp.

6. In a small bowl, whisk together soy sauce, hoisin sauce, sesame oil, and grated ginger.

7. Pour the sauce over the vegetables in the skillet and toss to coat evenly. Cook for an additional 2-3 minutes, allowing the flavors to meld.

8. Add the cooked quinoa to the vegetable mixture in the skillet, tossing to combine and heat through.

9. Garnish the quinoa and vegetable stir-fry with chopped green onions and sesame seeds, if desired.

10. Serve the stir-fry hot, and enjoy a flavorful and nutritious meal!

Salmon and Asparagus Bundle

Ingredients:

- 4 salmon filets (about 6 ounces each)
- Salt and black pepper to taste
- 1 tablespoon olive oil
- 1 bunch asparagus, trimmed
- 1 lemon, sliced
- 4 cloves garlic, minced

- 2 tablespoons fresh dill, chopped
- 2 tablespoons Dijon mustard
- 2 tablespoons honey
- 2 tablespoons soy sauce

Instructions:

1. Preheat the oven to 400°F (200°C).
2. Season the salmon filets with salt and black pepper. Set aside.
3. In a large bowl, toss the trimmed asparagus with olive oil, minced garlic, and salt.
4. Cut four large pieces of parchment paper, each about 12 inches square.
5. Place a portion of asparagus in the center of each parchment paper square.
6. Top each bed of asparagus with a salmon filet.
7. In a small bowl, whisk together Dijon mustard, honey, and soy sauce to create the glaze.
8. Brush each salmon filet with the glaze, and top with lemon slices.
9. Sprinkle fresh dill over each salmon filet.
10. Fold the parchment paper over the salmon and asparagus, creating a bundle. Roll and crimp the edges to seal.
11. Place the parchment bundles on a baking sheet.

12. Bake in the preheated oven for 15-20 minutes, depending on the thickness of the salmon, until the salmon is cooked through and flakes easily with a fork.
13. Carefully open the parchment bundles, allowing steam to escape. Be cautious, as the steam will be hot.
14. Serve the salmon and asparagus bundles directly in the parchment paper or transfer to plates.
15. Garnish with additional fresh dill and lemon slices if desired.

Lentil Soup with Greens

Ingredients:

- 1 cup dried green or brown lentils, rinsed and drained
- 1 onion, finely chopped
- 2 carrots, diced
- 2 celery stalks, diced
- 3 cloves garlic, minced
- 1 teaspoon ground cumin
- 1 teaspoon ground coriander
- 1/2 teaspoon smoked paprika
- 1 bay leaf

- 6 cups vegetable broth
- 1 can (14 ounces) diced tomatoes, undrained
- 4 cups fresh greens (spinach, kale, Swiss chard, or a mix), chopped
- Salt and black pepper to taste
- 2 tablespoons olive oil
- Lemon wedges (optional, for serving)

Instructions:

1. In a large soup pot, heat olive oil over medium heat.
2. Add chopped onions, carrots, and celery to the pot. Sauté for 5-7 minutes, or until the vegetables are softened.
3. Add minced garlic, ground cumin, ground coriander, and smoked paprika to the pot. Stir and cook for an additional 1-2 minutes until the spices are fragrant.
4. Pour in the rinsed lentils, vegetable broth, diced tomatoes (with their juice), and bay leaf. Bring the mixture to a boil.
5. Reduce the heat to low, cover the pot, and let the soup simmer for about 25-30 minutes or until the lentils are tender.

6. Stir in the chopped greens and cook for an additional 5-7 minutes until the greens are wilted.

7. Season the lentil soup with salt and black pepper to taste. Adjust the seasoning as needed.

8. Remove the bay leaf from the soup and discard.

9. Serve the lentil soup hot, optionally squeezing fresh lemon juice over each bowl for a burst of brightness.

10. Enjoy a comforting and nutritious bowl of Lentil Soup with Greens!

Turkey and Avocado Wrap

Ingredients:

- 1 pound cooked turkey breast, sliced
- 4 large whole wheat or spinach tortillas
- 1 large avocado, sliced
- 1 cup cherry tomatoes, halved
- 1/2 cup red onion, thinly sliced
- 1 cup fresh spinach leaves
- 1/4 cup mayonnaise
- 2 tablespoons Dijon mustard
- 1 tablespoon honey
- Salt and black pepper to taste

- Optional: Sliced cheese (cheddar, Swiss, or your choice)

Instructions:

1. In a small bowl, whisk together mayonnaise, Dijon mustard, honey, salt, and black pepper to create the dressing.
2. Lay out the tortillas on a clean surface.
3. Spread a generous layer of the dressing over each tortilla, leaving about an inch border around the edges.
4. Place a handful of fresh spinach leaves in the center of each tortilla, followed by sliced turkey, avocado slices, cherry tomatoes, and red onion.
5. If desired, add a layer of sliced cheese over the ingredients.
6. Fold in the sides of the tortilla and then roll it up tightly from the bottom to create a wrap.
7. Repeat the process for the remaining tortillas.
8. Optionally, you can secure each wrap with toothpicks or parchment paper.
9. Slice the wraps in half diagonally for easier serving.
10. Serve immediately and enjoy your delicious Turkey and Avocado Wraps!

Mushroom and Brown Rice Risotto

Ingredients:

- 1 cup brown rice
- 8 oz (about 225g) mushrooms, sliced (use a mix of varieties like cremini, shiitake, and oyster for depth of flavor)
- 1 onion, finely chopped
- 2 cloves garlic, minced
- 4 cups vegetable broth, kept warm
- 1 cup dry white wine
- 2 tablespoons olive oil
- 1 cup Parmesan cheese, grated
- 2 tablespoons unsalted butter
- Salt and black pepper to taste
- Fresh parsley, chopped (for garnish)

Instructions:

1. Rinse the brown rice under cold water and set it aside.
2. In a large, deep skillet or a wide saucepan, heat the olive oil over medium heat.
3. Add the chopped onion and sauté until it becomes translucent, about 3-4 minutes.
4. Stir in the minced garlic and cook for an additional 1-2 minutes until fragrant.

5. Add the sliced mushrooms to the pan and cook until they release their moisture and become golden brown, approximately 5-7 minutes.

6. Pour in the brown rice and stir to coat it in the oil and mix it with the mushrooms and onions. Toast the rice for about 2 minutes.

7. Deglaze the pan by pouring in the dry white wine. Stir constantly until most of the wine is absorbed.

8. Begin adding the warm vegetable broth, one ladle at a time, stirring frequently. Allow the liquid to be mostly absorbed before adding the next ladle of broth.

9. Continue this process until the brown rice is cooked and has a creamy consistency. This will take about 40-50 minutes. Adjust the heat to maintain a gentle simmer.

10. Once the rice is cooked, stir in the grated Parmesan cheese and butter. Season with salt and black pepper to taste.

11. Remove the risotto from heat, cover, and let it rest for a couple of minutes.

12. Serve the Mushroom and Brown Rice Risotto hot, garnished with fresh chopped parsley.

Vegetable and Quinoa Stuffed Peppers

Ingredients:

- 4 large bell peppers, halved and seeds removed
- 1 cup quinoa, rinsed and drained
- 2 cups vegetable broth
- 1 tablespoon olive oil
- 1 onion, finely chopped
- 2 cloves garlic, minced
- 1 zucchini, diced
- 1 carrot, grated
- 1 cup cherry tomatoes, halved
- 1 cup corn kernels (fresh, frozen, or canned)
- 1 teaspoon ground cumin
- 1 teaspoon paprika
- Salt and black pepper to taste
- 1 cup black beans, drained and rinsed
- 1 cup shredded cheese (cheddar, mozzarella, or your choice)
- Fresh cilantro or parsley for garnish (optional)
- Salsa or sour cream for serving (optional)

Instructions:

1. Preheat the oven to 375°F (190°C).
2. In a medium saucepan, combine quinoa and vegetable broth.

3. Bring to a boil, then reduce heat to low, cover, and simmer for about 15 minutes or until the quinoa is cooked and the liquid is absorbed. Fluff with a fork and set aside.

4. Heat olive oil in a large skillet over medium heat.

5. Add chopped onions and sauté for 3-4 minutes until they become translucent.

6. Stir in minced garlic, diced zucchini, and grated carrot. Cook for an additional 3-4 minutes until the vegetables are softened.

7. Add halved cherry tomatoes, corn kernels, ground cumin, paprika, salt, and black pepper to the skillet. Cook for another 3-4 minutes until the tomatoes release their juices.

8. Mix in the cooked quinoa and black beans, stirring until everything is well combined and heated through.

9. Arrange the halved bell peppers in a baking dish.

10. Spoon the quinoa and vegetable mixture into each bell pepper half, pressing down gently.

11. Sprinkle shredded cheese over the stuffed peppers.

12. Cover the baking dish with foil and bake in the preheated oven for 25-30 minutes, or until the peppers are tender.

13. If desired, uncover the dish for the last 5 minutes of baking to allow the cheese to melt and slightly brown.

14. Remove from the oven and let the stuffed peppers cool for a few minutes.

15. Garnish with fresh cilantro or parsley if desired.

16. Serve the Vegetable and Quinoa Stuffed Peppers with salsa or sour cream on the side, if you like.

Baked Cod with Lemon Dill Sauce

Ingredients:

For Baked Cod:

- 4 cod filets (about 6 ounces each)
- Salt and black pepper to taste
- 2 tablespoons olive oil
- 2 tablespoons fresh lemon juice
- 2 teaspoons garlic powder
- 1 teaspoon dried oregano
- 1 teaspoon paprika
- Lemon slices for garnish

For Lemon Dill Sauce:

- 1/2 cup plain Greek yogurt
- 2 tablespoons mayonnaise
- 1 tablespoon fresh dill, chopped
- 1 tablespoon fresh lemon juice
- 1 teaspoon Dijon mustard
- Salt and black pepper to taste

Instructions:

1. Preheat the oven to 400°F (200°C).

2. Pat the cod filets dry with paper towels and place them on a baking sheet lined with parchment paper.

3. In a small bowl, mix together olive oil, fresh lemon juice, garlic powder, dried oregano, paprika, salt, and black pepper.

4. Brush the cod filets with the lemon and spice mixture, ensuring they are well coated on all sides.

5. Bake in the preheated oven for 12-15 minutes or until the cod is opaque and easily flakes with a fork.

6. While the cod is baking, prepare the Lemon Dill Sauce.

7. In a bowl, combine Greek yogurt, mayonnaise, chopped dill, fresh lemon juice, Dijon mustard, salt, and black pepper. Mix until well combined.

8. Once the cod is done, remove it from the oven and let it rest for a few minutes.

9. Serve the baked cod filets with a drizzle of Lemon Dill Sauce on top.

10. Garnish with additional fresh dill and lemon slices.

11. Enjoy your flavorful and light Baked Cod with Lemon Dill Sauce!

Chickpea and Spinach Curry

Ingredients:

- 2 tablespoons vegetable oil
- 1 large onion, finely chopped
- 3 cloves garlic, minced
- 1 tablespoon fresh ginger, grated
- 1 tablespoon curry powder
- 1 teaspoon ground cumin
- 1 teaspoon ground coriander
- 1 teaspoon turmeric
- 1/2 teaspoon cayenne pepper (adjust to taste)
- 1 can (15 ounces) chickpeas, drained and rinsed

- 1 can (14 ounces) diced tomatoes
- 1 can (14 ounces) coconut milk
- 1 large bunch fresh spinach, washed and chopped
- Salt and black pepper to taste
- Fresh cilantro, chopped (for garnish)
- Cooked rice or naan bread (for serving)

Instructions:

1. In a large skillet or pot, heat the vegetable oil over medium heat.
2. Add the chopped onion and sauté until it becomes soft and translucent, about 5 minutes.
3. Stir in the minced garlic and grated ginger, cooking for an additional 1-2 minutes until fragrant.
4. Add the curry powder, ground cumin, ground coriander, turmeric, and cayenne pepper to the skillet. Stir well to coat the onions with the spices.
5. Pour in the diced tomatoes (with their juice) and chickpeas. Cook for 5 minutes, allowing the flavors to meld.

6. Add the coconut milk to the skillet, stirring to combine. Bring the mixture to a simmer, then reduce the heat to low.

7. Fold in the chopped spinach and cook until it wilts, about 3-5 minutes.

8. Season the chickpea and spinach curry with salt and black pepper to taste. Adjust the seasoning as needed.

9. Simmer the curry for an additional 5-10 minutes to allow the flavors to develop.

10. Serve the chickpea and spinach curry over cooked rice or with naan bread.

11. Garnish with chopped fresh cilantro.

12. Enjoy a hearty and flavorful Chickpea and Spinach Curry!

Caprese Salad with Grilled Chicken

For Grilled Chicken:

- 4 boneless, skinless chicken breasts
- Salt and black pepper to taste
- 2 tablespoons olive oil
- 1 teaspoon dried oregano
- 1 teaspoon garlic powder
- 1 teaspoon paprika

For Caprese Salad:

- 4 large tomatoes, sliced
- 1 pound fresh mozzarella cheese, sliced
- Fresh basil leaves
- Balsamic glaze (store-bought or homemade)
- Salt and black pepper to taste
- Extra virgin olive oil (optional, for drizzling)

Instructions:

Grilled Chicken:

1. Preheat the grill to medium-high heat.
2. Season the chicken breasts with salt, black pepper, dried oregano, garlic powder, and paprika. Drizzle with olive oil and rub the seasonings into the chicken.
3. Grill the chicken breasts for about 6-8 minutes per side or until the internal temperature reaches 165°F (74°C). Cooking time may vary depending on the thickness of the chicken. Once cooked, let the chicken rest for a few minutes before slicing it into strips.

Caprese Salad:

1. On a serving platter, alternate slices of tomatoes, fresh mozzarella, and basil leaves, creating a visually appealing pattern.

2. Arrange the grilled chicken strips on top of the Caprese salad.

3. Drizzle balsamic glaze over the salad. If you don't have balsamic glaze, you can mix balsamic vinegar with a bit of honey or maple syrup and reduce it on the stovetop until it thickens.

4. Season the salad with salt and black pepper to taste.

5. Optional: Drizzle extra virgin olive oil over the salad for added richness.

6. Garnish with additional fresh basil leaves.

7. Serve the Caprese Salad with Grilled Chicken immediately and enjoy the delightful combination of flavors!

Sweet Potato and Black Bean Bowl

Ingredients:

- 2 medium-sized sweet potatoes, peeled and diced
- 1 can (15 oz) black beans, drained and rinsed
- 1 cup cooked quinoa
- 1 red bell pepper, diced
- 1/2 red onion, finely chopped
- 1 cup corn kernels (fresh or frozen)

- 1 avocado, sliced
- 1/4 cup fresh cilantro, chopped
- 2 tablespoons olive oil
- 1 teaspoon ground cumin
- 1 teaspoon chili powder
- 1/2 teaspoon paprika
- Salt and pepper to taste
- Lime wedges for serving

Instructions:

1. Preheat the oven to 400°F (200°C).

2. In a large bowl, toss the diced sweet potatoes with 1 tablespoon of olive oil, ground cumin, chili powder, paprika, salt, and pepper until evenly coated. Spread the sweet potatoes on a baking sheet lined with parchment paper and roast for 20-25 minutes or until they are tender and slightly crispy.

3. While the sweet potatoes are roasting, heat the remaining olive oil in a skillet over medium heat. Add the diced red bell pepper, red onion, and corn kernels. Sauté for 5-7 minutes or until the vegetables are tender.

4. Add the black beans to the skillet and cook for an additional 2-3 minutes until heated through.

5. In a large bowl, combine the roasted sweet potatoes, sautéed vegetable and bean mixture, and cooked quinoa. Toss everything together until well mixed.

6. Divide the mixture into serving bowls. Top each bowl with sliced avocado and sprinkle with fresh cilantro.

7. Serve the sweet potato and black bean bowl with lime wedges on the side for a burst of citrus flavor.

Broccoli and Chicken Stir-Fry

Ingredients:

- 1 lb (about 450g) boneless, skinless chicken breasts, thinly sliced
- 4 cups broccoli florets
- 1 red bell pepper, thinly sliced
- 1 carrot, julienned
- 3 cloves garlic, minced
- 1 tablespoon fresh ginger, grated
- 1/4 cup soy sauce
- 2 tablespoons oyster sauce
- 1 tablespoon sesame oil
- 2 tablespoons vegetable oil (for cooking)

- 2 tablespoons cornstarch
- 1/4 cup water
- Cooked rice for serving

Instructions:

1. In a small bowl, mix the soy sauce, oyster sauce, sesame oil, and cornstarch. Stir until the cornstarch is dissolved. This will be your stir-fry sauce.

2. In a large skillet or wok, heat 1 tablespoon of vegetable oil over medium-high heat. Add the sliced chicken and stir-fry until it's fully cooked and slightly browned. Remove the chicken from the skillet and set it aside.

3. In the same skillet, add another tablespoon of vegetable oil. Stir in the minced garlic and grated ginger, cooking for about 30 seconds until fragrant.

4. Add the broccoli, red bell pepper, and julienned carrot to the skillet. Stir-fry the vegetables for 3-5 minutes or until they are tender-crisp.

5. Return the cooked chicken to the skillet with the vegetables. Pour the stir-fry sauce over the chicken and vegetables.

6. Toss everything together to coat evenly. Cook for an additional 2-3 minutes until the sauce thickens.

7. If needed, add 1/4 cup of water to the skillet to adjust the consistency of the sauce.

8. Serve the broccoli and chicken stir-fry over cooked rice. Garnish with sesame seeds or chopped green onions if desired.

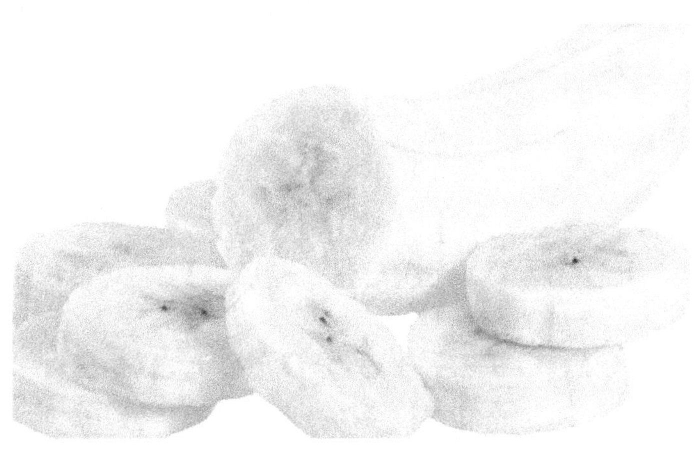

"I trust in my body's ability to heal, and I am surrounded by a supportive network."

"Each nutrient-rich meal I enjoy is a step towards better health and well-being."

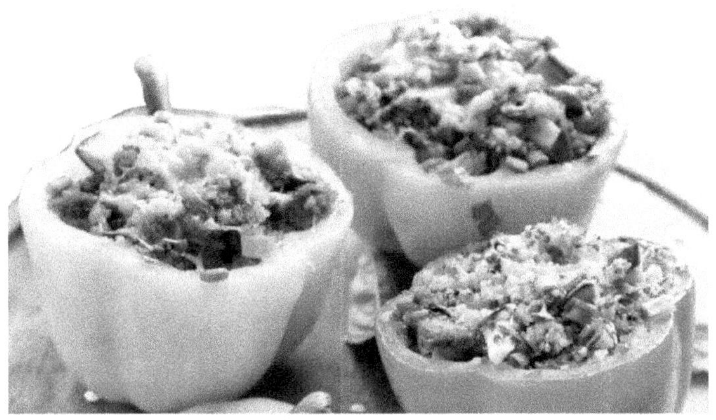

Baked Herb-Crusted Chicken

Ingredients:

- 4 boneless, skinless chicken breasts
- 1 cup breadcrumbs
- 1/2 cup grated Parmesan cheese
- 2 tablespoons fresh parsley, chopped
- 1 teaspoon dried thyme
- 1 teaspoon dried rosemary
- 1 teaspoon dried oregano
- 1/2 teaspoon garlic powder
- Salt and pepper to taste
- 1/4 cup olive oil

Instructions:

1. Preheat your oven to 400°F (200°C) and lightly grease a baking dish.

2. In a bowl, mix together breadcrumbs, Parmesan cheese, chopped parsley, dried thyme, dried rosemary, dried oregano, garlic powder, salt, and pepper. This is your herb crust mixture.

3. Brush each chicken breast with olive oil, ensuring they are well-coated.

4. Dredge each chicken breast in the herb crust mixture, pressing it onto the chicken to adhere.

5. Place the coated chicken breasts in the prepared baking dish.

6. If you have any remaining herb crust mixture, sprinkle it evenly over the chicken breasts.

7. Bake in the preheated oven for 25-30 minutes or until the chicken is cooked through and the crust is golden brown and crispy.

8. To ensure the chicken is fully cooked, use a meat thermometer to check that the internal temperature reaches 165°F (74°C).

9. Once done, remove the chicken from the oven and let it rest for a few minutes before serving.

Quinoa and Vegetable Stuffed Bell Peppers

Ingredients:

- 4 large bell peppers, any color
- 1 cup quinoa, rinsed
- 2 cups vegetable broth or water
- 1 tablespoon olive oil
- 1 onion, finely chopped
- 2 cloves garlic, minced
- 1 zucchini, diced
- 1 carrot, diced
- 1 cup cherry tomatoes, halved
- 1 cup corn kernels (fresh or frozen)
- 1 teaspoon ground cumin
- 1 teaspoon paprika
- Salt and pepper to taste
- 1 cup black beans, cooked (canned is fine)
- 1 cup shredded cheese (cheddar, mozzarella, or your choice)

Instructions:

1. Preheat your oven to 375°F (190°C).
2. Cut the tops off the bell peppers and remove the seeds and membranes.

3. If needed, trim the bottoms slightly to help them stand upright in the baking dish.

4. In a medium saucepan, combine quinoa and vegetable broth (or water). Bring to a boil, then reduce the heat, cover, and simmer for about 15 minutes or until the quinoa is cooked and the liquid is absorbed.

5. In a large skillet, heat olive oil over medium heat. Add chopped onion and garlic, sauté until softened.

6. Add diced zucchini, carrots, cherry tomatoes, and corn to the skillet. Cook for about 5-7 minutes until the vegetables are tender.

7. Stir in ground cumin, paprika, salt, and pepper. Mix well.

8. Add cooked quinoa and black beans to the skillet. Stir until all the ingredients are combined and heated through.

9. Place the bell peppers in a baking dish. Spoon the quinoa and vegetable mixture into each pepper until they are fully stuffed.

10. Top each stuffed pepper with shredded cheese.

11. Cover the baking dish with foil and bake in the preheated oven for 25-30 minutes, or until the peppers are tender.

12. If you prefer a crispy cheese topping, uncover the dish for the last 5-10 minutes of baking.

13. Remove from the oven and let it cool for a few minutes before serving.

Salmon with Roasted Brussels Sprouts

Ingredients:

- 4 salmon filets
- 1 lb Brussels sprouts, trimmed and halved
- 2 tablespoons olive oil
- 1 tablespoon Dijon mustard
- 2 tablespoons honey
- 2 cloves garlic, minced
- 1 teaspoon dried thyme
- Salt and pepper to taste
- Lemon wedges for serving

Instructions:

1. Preheat your oven to 400°F (200°C).

2. In a large bowl, toss Brussels sprouts with 1 tablespoon of olive oil, salt, and pepper. Spread them evenly on a baking sheet.

3. Roast Brussels sprouts in the preheated oven for 20-25 minutes or until they are golden brown and crispy on the edges. Stir them halfway through the roasting time for even cooking.

4. While the Brussels sprouts are roasting, prepare the salmon. In a small bowl, whisk together Dijon mustard, honey, minced garlic, dried thyme, salt, and pepper.

5. Place the salmon filets on a separate baking sheet lined with parchment paper or aluminum foil.

6. Brush the salmon filets with the Dijon-honey mixture, making sure they are well coated.

7. Once the Brussels sprouts are done roasting, increase the oven temperature to 425°F (220°C).

8. Place the salmon in the oven and bake for 12-15 minutes or until the salmon is cooked through and flakes easily with a fork.

9. While the salmon is baking, drizzle the remaining olive oil over the roasted Brussels sprouts for added flavor.

10. Serve the salmon filets on a plate alongside the roasted Brussels sprouts.

11. Garnish with lemon wedges for a fresh, citrusy touch.

Vegetarian Lentil Stew

Ingredients:

- 1 cup dry green or brown lentils, rinsed and drained
- 1 large onion, finely chopped
- 3 carrots, peeled and diced
- 3 celery stalks, diced
- 4 cloves garlic, minced
- 1 can (14 oz) diced tomatoes
- 1 can (6 oz) tomato paste
- 6 cups vegetable broth
- 2 teaspoons ground cumin
- 1 teaspoon ground coriander
- 1 teaspoon smoked paprika
- 1 teaspoon dried thyme
- 1 bay leaf
- Salt and pepper to taste
- 2 tablespoons olive oil
- 2 cups chopped kale or spinach (optional)
- Fresh parsley for garnish

Instructions:

1. In a large pot, heat olive oil over medium heat. Add chopped onion, carrots, and celery. Sauté for about 5 minutes until the vegetables are softened.

2. Add minced garlic and continue to sauté for another minute until fragrant.

3. Stir in ground cumin, ground coriander, smoked paprika, and dried thyme. Cook for an additional 2 minutes to enhance the flavors.

4. Add rinsed lentils, diced tomatoes, tomato paste, vegetable broth, bay leaf, salt, and pepper to the pot. Stir well to combine.

5. Bring the stew to a boil, then reduce the heat to low, cover, and simmer for about 25-30 minutes or until the lentils are tender.

6. If using, add chopped kale or spinach to the stew during the last 5 minutes of cooking, allowing it to wilt.

7. Taste and adjust the seasoning if needed. Remove the bay leaf before serving.

8. Ladle the vegetarian lentil stew into bowls and garnish with fresh parsley.

9. Serve hot and enjoy your hearty and nutritious Vegetarian Lentil Stew!

Grilled Turkey Burger with Sweet Potato Fries

Ingredients for Turkey Burger:

- 1 lb ground turkey
- 1/2 cup breadcrumbs
- 1/4 cup grated Parmesan cheese
- 1/4 cup finely chopped onion
- 1 clove garlic, minced
- 1 tablespoon Worcestershire sauce
- 1 teaspoon dried oregano
- Salt and pepper to taste
- Olive oil for grilling
- Whole wheat burger buns

Ingredients for Sweet Potato Fries:

- 2 large sweet potatoes, peeled and cut into matchsticks
- 2 tablespoons olive oil
- 1 teaspoon smoked paprika
- 1/2 teaspoon garlic powder
- 1/2 teaspoon cumin
- Salt and pepper to taste

Instructions for Turkey Burger:

1. In a large bowl, combine ground turkey, breadcrumbs, Parmesan cheese, chopped onion, minced garlic, Worcestershire sauce, dried oregano, salt, and pepper. Mix until well combined.
2. Divide the turkey mixture into equal portions and shape them into burger patties.
3. Preheat your grill or grill pan over medium-high heat.
4. Brush each turkey patty with olive oil to prevent sticking.
5. Grill the turkey burgers for about 5-7 minutes per side, or until they are fully cooked and have an internal temperature of 165°F (74°C).
6. Toast the whole wheat burger buns on the grill for a minute or two.
7. Assemble your grilled turkey burgers on the toasted buns and add your favorite toppings like lettuce, tomato, and condiments.

Instructions for Sweet Potato Fries:

1. Preheat your oven to 425°F (220°C).

2. In a large bowl, toss sweet potato matchsticks with olive oil, smoked paprika, garlic powder, cumin, salt, and pepper until evenly coated.

3. Spread the sweet potato fries in a single layer on a baking sheet lined with parchment paper.

4. Bake in the preheated oven for 20-25 minutes, flipping the fries halfway through, or until they are golden and crispy.

5. Remove the sweet potato fries from the oven and season with additional salt if needed.

Mushroom and Spinach Frittata

Ingredients:

- 8 large eggs
- 1/2 cup milk
- Salt and pepper to taste
- 2 tablespoons olive oil
- 1 small onion, finely chopped
- 8 oz mushrooms, sliced
- 2 cups fresh spinach, chopped
- 1 cup shredded Gruyere or your favorite cheese
- 1 teaspoon dried thyme (optional)
- Fresh herbs (such as parsley or chives) for garnish

Instructions:

1. Preheat your oven to 375°F (190°C).

2. In a bowl, whisk together eggs, milk, salt, and pepper. Set aside.

3. Heat olive oil in a large oven-safe skillet over medium heat.

4. Add chopped onion to the skillet and sauté for 2-3 minutes until softened.

5. Add sliced mushrooms to the skillet and cook for another 5-7 minutes until they release their moisture and become golden brown.

6. Stir in chopped spinach and cook for 2-3 minutes until wilted.

7. If using, add dried thyme for additional flavor.

8. Pour the egg mixture over the vegetables in the skillet. Stir gently to ensure the ingredients are evenly distributed.

9. Sprinkle shredded cheese evenly over the top of the frittata.

10. Cook on the stovetop for 3-4 minutes without stirring to let the edges set.

11. Transfer the skillet to the preheated oven and bake for 15-20 minutes or until the frittata is set in the center and the top is golden brown.

12. Remove from the oven and let it cool for a few minutes.

13. Garnish with fresh herbs.

14. Slice the Mushroom and Spinach Frittata into wedges and serve.

Cauliflower and Chickpea Curry

Ingredients:

- 1 medium cauliflower, cut into florets
- 1 can (15 oz) chickpeas, drained and rinsed
- 1 large onion, finely chopped
- 3 cloves garlic, minced
- 1 tablespoon ginger, grated
- 1 can (14 oz) diced tomatoes
- 1 can (14 oz) coconut milk
- 2 tablespoons tomato paste
- 2 tablespoons curry powder
- 1 teaspoon ground cumin
- 1 teaspoon ground coriander
- 1/2 teaspoon turmeric
- 1/2 teaspoon cayenne pepper (adjust to taste for spice level)
- Salt and pepper to taste
- 2 tablespoons vegetable oil

- Fresh cilantro for garnish
- Cooked rice or naan for serving

Instructions:

1. Heat vegetable oil in a large pot or deep skillet over medium heat.

2. Add chopped onion and cook until softened, about 5 minutes.

3. Stir in minced garlic and grated ginger, cooking for an additional 1-2 minutes until fragrant.

4. Add curry powder, ground cumin, ground coriander, turmeric, cayenne pepper, salt, and pepper. Stir well to coat the onions, garlic, and ginger with the spices.

5. Add tomato paste to the pot, stirring to combine with the spices.

6. Pour in the diced tomatoes (with their juices) and coconut milk. Bring the mixture to a simmer.

7. Add cauliflower florets and chickpeas to the pot. Stir to coat them in the curry sauce.

8. Cover the pot and simmer for 20-25 minutes, or until the cauliflower is tender.

9. Taste and adjust the seasoning if needed.

10. Serve the Cauliflower and Chickpea Curry over cooked rice or with naan.

11. Garnish with fresh cilantro before serving.

Herb-Roasted Cod with Quinoa Pilaf

Ingredients for Herb-Roasted Cod:

- 4 cod filets (about 6 oz each)
- 2 tablespoons olive oil
- 1 tablespoon fresh lemon juice
- 2 cloves garlic, minced
- 1 teaspoon dried thyme
- 1 teaspoon dried rosemary
- Salt and pepper to taste
- Lemon wedges for serving

Ingredients for Quinoa Pilaf:

- 1 cup quinoa, rinsed
- 2 cups vegetable broth or water
- 1 tablespoon olive oil
- 1 small onion, finely chopped
- 2 carrots, diced
- 1 zucchini, diced
- 1/4 cup pine nuts (optional)
- 1 teaspoon ground cumin
- Salt and pepper to taste

- Fresh parsley for garnish

Instructions for Herb-Roasted Cod:

1. Preheat your oven to 400°F (200°C).
2. In a small bowl, mix together olive oil, fresh lemon juice, minced garlic, dried thyme, dried rosemary, salt, and pepper.
3. Place the cod filets on a baking sheet lined with parchment paper.
4. Brush the cod filets with the herb mixture, ensuring they are well-coated.
5. Roast in the preheated oven for 12-15 minutes, or until the cod is opaque and flakes easily with a fork.
6. While the cod is roasting, prepare the quinoa pilaf.

Instructions for Quinoa Pilaf:

1. In a medium saucepan, combine quinoa and vegetable broth (or water). Bring to a boil, then reduce heat, cover, and simmer for about 15 minutes or until the quinoa is cooked and the liquid is absorbed.
2. In a separate skillet, heat olive oil over medium heat.

3. Add chopped onion, diced carrots, and diced zucchini to the skillet. Sauté for about 5-7 minutes until the vegetables are tender.

4. If using, add pine nuts to the skillet and toast for a few minutes until they are golden brown.

5. Stir in ground cumin, salt, and pepper. Mix well.

6. Add the cooked quinoa to the skillet with the sautéed vegetables and pine nuts. Stir to combine.

7. Garnish the quinoa pilaf with fresh parsley.

Zucchini Noodles with Pesto and Grilled Chicken

Ingredients:

For Zucchini Noodles:

- 4 medium-sized zucchinis, spiralized
- 1 tablespoon olive oil
- Salt and pepper to taste

For Pesto Sauce:

- 2 cups fresh basil leaves
- 1/2 cup grated Parmesan cheese
- 1/2 cup pine nuts or walnuts
- 2 cloves garlic, peeled
- 1/2 cup extra-virgin olive oil

- Salt and pepper to taste

- Juice of 1 lemon

For Grilled Chicken:

- 2 boneless, skinless chicken breasts

- 1 tablespoon olive oil

- Salt and pepper to taste

Instructions:

For Zucchini Noodles:

1. Spiralize the zucchinis to create zucchini noodles. If you don't have a spiralizer, you can use a vegetable peeler to create ribbon-like strands.

2. Heat olive oil in a large pan over medium heat. Add the zucchini noodles, season with salt and pepper, and sauté for 3-5 minutes or until just tender. Be careful not to overcook; you want the noodles to have a slight crunch.

For Pesto Sauce:

1. In a food processor, combine fresh basil, grated Parmesan cheese, pine nuts or walnuts, and peeled garlic.

2. Pulse until the ingredients are finely chopped.

3. With the food processor running, slowly pour in the extra-virgin olive oil until the mixture reaches a smooth and creamy consistency.

4. Season the pesto with salt, pepper, and the juice of one lemon. Adjust the seasoning to your taste.

For Grilled Chicken:

1. Preheat a grill or grill pan over medium-high heat.

2. Rub the chicken breasts with olive oil and season with salt and pepper.

3. Grill the chicken for 6-8 minutes per side or until fully cooked and the internal temperature reaches 165°F (74°C).

4. Let the grilled chicken rest for a few minutes before slicing it into strips.

To Serve:

1. Toss the sautéed zucchini noodles with a generous amount of pesto sauce.

2. Top the zucchini noodles with sliced grilled chicken.

3. Optionally, garnish with additional grated Parmesan cheese and fresh basil leaves.

4. Serve immediately and enjoy this light and flavorful zucchini noodle dish with pesto and grilled chicken.

Stuffed Acorn Squash with Turkey and Cranberries

Ingredients:

- 2 acorn squashes, halved and seeds removed
- 1 pound ground turkey
- 1 tablespoon olive oil
- 1 onion, finely chopped
- 2 cloves garlic, minced
- 1 teaspoon dried sage
- 1 teaspoon dried thyme
- Salt and pepper to taste
- 1 cup cooked quinoa or wild rice
- 1/2 cup dried cranberries
- 1/2 cup chopped pecans or walnuts
- 1/4 cup fresh parsley, chopped
- 1/2 cup feta cheese, crumbled (optional)
- Maple syrup for drizzling (optional)

Instructions:

1. Preheat the oven to 400°F (200°C).

2. Place the acorn squash halves on a baking sheet, cut side up. Drizzle with olive oil and sprinkle with salt and pepper. Roast in the preheated oven for 30-35 minutes or until the squash is tender.

3. While the squash is roasting, prepare the filling. In a large skillet, heat olive oil over medium heat.

4. Add chopped onion and minced garlic to the skillet. Sauté until the onion is softened.

5. Add ground turkey to the skillet, breaking it apart with a spoon. Cook until browned.

6. Season the turkey with dried sage, dried thyme, salt, and pepper. Stir well to combine.

7. In a large mixing bowl, combine the cooked ground turkey with cooked quinoa or wild rice, dried cranberries, chopped nuts, fresh parsley, and crumbled feta cheese if using. Mix until well combined.

8. Once the acorn squash halves are roasted, fill each half with the turkey and quinoa mixture.

9. Optionally, drizzle maple syrup over the stuffed squash for added sweetness.

10. Return the stuffed acorn squash to the oven and bake for an additional 10-15 minutes or until heated through.

11. Serve the stuffed acorn squash with turkey and cranberries hot from the oven.

Spaghetti Squash Primavera

Ingredients:

- 1 medium-sized spaghetti squash
- 2 tablespoons olive oil
- 1 onion, thinly sliced
- 2 bell peppers, thinly sliced (use a mix of colors for visual appeal)
- 1 zucchini, thinly sliced
- 1 cup cherry tomatoes, halved
- 2 cloves garlic, minced
- Salt and pepper to taste
- 1/2 teaspoon dried oregano
- 1/2 teaspoon dried basil
- 1/4 teaspoon red pepper flakes (optional)
- Grated Parmesan cheese for garnish
- Fresh basil or parsley for garnish

Instructions:

1. Preheat the oven to 400°F (200°C).

2. Cut the spaghetti squash in half lengthwise and scoop out the seeds. Place the squash halves on a baking sheet, cut side up.

3. Drizzle olive oil over the cut sides of the spaghetti squash and season with salt and pepper.

4. Roast the spaghetti squash in the preheated oven for 40-50 minutes or until the flesh is tender and easily pierced with a fork.

5. While the spaghetti squash is roasting, prepare the vegetables. In a large skillet, heat olive oil over medium heat.

6. Add thinly sliced onion, bell peppers, and zucchini to the skillet. Sauté for 5-7 minutes or until the vegetables are tender-crisp.

7. Add minced garlic to the skillet and sauté for an additional 1-2 minutes until fragrant.

8. Stir in halved cherry tomatoes, dried oregano, dried basil, and red pepper flakes if using. Cook for another 2-3 minutes until the tomatoes are slightly softened.

9. Once the spaghetti squash is done roasting, use a fork to scrape the flesh into spaghetti-like strands.

10. Add the spaghetti squash strands to the skillet with the sautéed vegetables. Toss everything together until well combined.

11. Season the dish with additional salt and pepper to taste.

12. Garnish the Spaghetti Squash Primavera with grated Parmesan cheese and fresh basil or parsley.

13. Serve immediately and enjoy this light and flavorful vegetable-packed dish.

Baked Eggplant Parmesan

Ingredients:

- 2 medium-sized eggplants, sliced into 1/2-inch rounds
- Salt, for sweating the eggplant
- 2 cups marinara sauce
- 1 cup breadcrumbs (preferably Italian-style)
- 1 cup grated Parmesan cheese
- 2 cups shredded mozzarella cheese
- 2 large eggs
- 1/4 cup fresh basil, chopped
- 1/4 cup fresh parsley, chopped
- 1/2 teaspoon dried oregano

- 1/2 teaspoon dried thyme
- Olive oil, for brushing the eggplant slices
- Cooking spray, for greasing the baking sheet

Instructions:

1. Preheat the oven to 375°F (190°C). Grease a baking sheet with cooking spray.

2. Slice the eggplants into rounds, about 1/2 inch thick. Place the slices in a colander, sprinkle with salt, and let them sit for 30 minutes. This helps draw out excess moisture from the eggplant.

3. After 30 minutes, rinse the eggplant slices under cold water and pat them dry with a clean kitchen towel.

4. In a shallow dish, beat the eggs.

5. In another dish, combine breadcrumbs, grated Parmesan, dried oregano, dried thyme, and half of the chopped basil and parsley.

6. Dip each eggplant slice into the beaten eggs, allowing excess to drip off, and then coat it with the breadcrumb mixture, pressing gently to adhere.

7. Place the coated eggplant slices on the prepared baking sheet. Brush each slice with olive oil.

8. Bake in the preheated oven for 20-25 minutes or until the eggplant is golden and crispy.

9. In a baking dish, spread a thin layer of marinara sauce.

10. Arrange a layer of baked eggplant slices over the sauce.

11. Sprinkle a portion of shredded mozzarella over the eggplant.

12. Repeat the layers until you've used all the eggplant, finishing with a layer of marinara sauce and a generous topping of mozzarella.

13. Bake in the oven for an additional 25-30 minutes or until the cheese is melted and bubbly.

14. Garnish with the remaining chopped basil and parsley.

15. Let it rest for a few minutes before serving.

CHAPTER 6: SNACK RECIPES

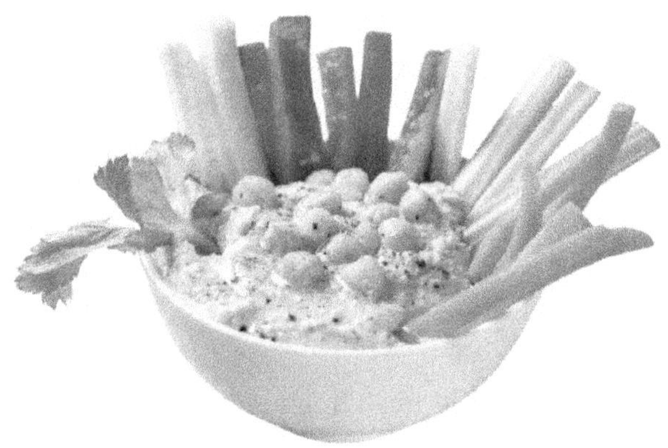

Greek Yogurt with Berries

Ingredients:

- 1 cup Greek yogurt
- 1/2 cup mixed berries (strawberries, blueberries, raspberries)
- 1 tablespoon honey or maple syrup (optional)
- 2 tablespoons granola
- Fresh mint leaves for garnish (optional)

Instructions:

1. In a serving bowl or glass, spoon Greek yogurt to create a smooth base.

2. Wash and prepare the mixed berries. You can leave them whole or cut larger berries into bite-sized pieces.

3. Arrange the mixed berries on top of the Greek yogurt.

4. Optionally, drizzle honey or maple syrup over the yogurt and berries for added sweetness.

5. Sprinkle granola evenly over the mixture. This adds a delightful crunch.

6. Garnish with fresh mint leaves for a burst of freshness (optional).

7. Serve the Greek yogurt with berries immediately and enjoy a simple, nutritious, and delicious snack or breakfast.

Hummus and Veggie Sticks

Ingredients:

For Hummus:

- 1 can (15 oz) chickpeas (garbanzo beans), drained and rinsed
- 1/4 cup tahini
- 1/4 cup extra-virgin olive oil
- 2 tablespoons lemon juice
- 2 cloves garlic, minced

- 1/2 teaspoon ground cumin
- Salt and pepper to taste
- 2-3 tablespoons water (as needed for consistency)

For Veggie Sticks:

- Carrot sticks
- Cucumber sticks
- Bell pepper strips (assorted colors)
- Cherry tomatoes, halved
- Celery sticks

Instructions:

For Hummus:

1. In a food processor, combine chickpeas, tahini, olive oil, lemon juice, minced garlic, ground cumin, salt, and pepper.
2. Blend the ingredients until smooth, scraping down the sides of the processor as needed.
3. If the hummus is too thick, add water, one tablespoon at a time, until you reach your desired consistency.
4. Taste and adjust the seasoning if needed.
5. Transfer the hummus to a serving bowl.

For Veggie Sticks:

1. Wash and prepare the vegetables. Peel and cut carrots and cucumbers into sticks. Slice bell peppers into strips.
2. Arrange the veggie sticks on a serving platter.
3. Optionally, place the hummus bowl in the center of the platter or use a separate dipping bowl.
4. Serve the hummus and veggie sticks together as a healthy and satisfying snack or appetizer.

Almond Butter and Banana Slices

Ingredients:

- 2 ripe bananas, peeled and sliced
- 1/4 cup almond butter (or any nut butter of your choice)
- 1-2 tablespoons honey or maple syrup (optional)
- 2 tablespoons chopped almonds (optional)

Instructions:

1. Peel and slice the ripe bananas into rounds.
2. In a small microwave-safe bowl, gently warm the almond butter for about 15-20 seconds until it becomes smooth and slightly runny.
3. Arrange the banana slices on a serving plate.

4. Drizzle the warmed almond butter over the banana slices. Optionally, drizzle honey or maple syrup for added sweetness.

5. If desired, sprinkle chopped almonds over the almond butter-covered banana slices for extra crunch.

6. Serve the almond butter and banana slices immediately and enjoy this simple and nutritious snack.

Mixed Nuts and Dried Fruits

Ingredients:

- 1 cup mixed nuts (almonds, walnuts, cashews, pistachios)
- 1/2 cup dried cranberries
- 1/2 cup dried apricots, chopped
- 1/2 cup dried figs, sliced
- 1/4 cup pumpkin seeds (optional)
- 1/4 cup dark chocolate chips (optional)

Instructions:

1. In a dry skillet over medium heat, toast the mixed nuts for 3-5 minutes, stirring frequently until they become fragrant. Be careful not to burn them.

2. Once toasted, remove the nuts from the skillet and let them cool.

3. In a mixing bowl, combine the toasted mixed nuts with dried cranberries, chopped dried apricots, sliced dried figs, pumpkin seeds (if using), and dark chocolate chips (if using).

4. Toss the ingredients together until well mixed.

5. Transfer the mixed nuts and dried fruits to an airtight container for storage.

6. Serve as a snack, trail mix, or a topping for yogurt or oatmeal.

Homemade Trail Mix

Ingredients:

- 1 cup almonds
- 1 cup walnuts
- 1 cup cashews
- 1 cup dried cranberries
- 1 cup raisins
- 1 cup dark chocolate chips
- 1 cup pretzel sticks
- 1 cup banana chips

Instructions:

1. In a dry skillet over medium heat, toast the almonds, walnuts, and cashews for 3-5 minutes, stirring frequently until they become fragrant. Be cautious not to burn them.
2. Once toasted, remove the nuts from the skillet and let them cool.
3. In a large mixing bowl, combine the toasted almonds, walnuts, and cashews with dried cranberries, raisins, dark chocolate chips, pretzel sticks, and banana chips.
4. Toss the ingredients together until well mixed.
5. Transfer the homemade trail mix to an airtight container for storage.
6. Shake the container to mix the ingredients before serving.
7. Portion the trail mix into snack-sized bags for convenient and portable servings.

Cottage Cheese with Pineapple

Ingredients:

- 1 cup cottage cheese
- 1 cup fresh pineapple chunks (or canned pineapple tidbits, drained)

- 1 tablespoon honey (optional)
- 2 tablespoons chopped fresh mint (optional)

Instructions:

1. In a serving bowl, scoop out the cottage cheese.
2. Add fresh pineapple chunks on top of the cottage cheese.
3. Optionally, drizzle honey over the cottage cheese and pineapple for added sweetness.
4. Garnish with chopped fresh mint if desired.
5. Gently mix the ingredients together to combine flavors.
6. Serve the Cottage Cheese with Pineapple immediately and enjoy this refreshing and protein-packed snack.

Whole Grain Toast with Avocado

Ingredients:

- 2 slices whole grain bread
- 1 ripe avocado
- 1 tablespoon olive oil
- Salt and pepper to taste
- Red pepper flakes (optional)
- Lemon wedges for serving (optional)
- Fresh cilantro or parsley for garnish (optional)

Instructions:

1. Toast the whole grain bread slices to your desired level of crispiness.
2. While the bread is toasting, cut the avocado in half and remove the pit. Scoop out the avocado flesh into a bowl.
3. Mash the avocado with a fork until it reaches your preferred consistency.
4. Drizzle olive oil over the mashed avocado and season with salt and pepper. Mix well.
5. Once the toast is ready, spread the mashed avocado evenly over each slice.
6. Optionally, sprinkle red pepper flakes on top for a hint of heat.
7. Garnish with fresh cilantro or parsley if desired.
8. Serve the Whole Grain Toast with Avocado immediately, with lemon wedges on the side if you like.

Edamame Pods

Ingredients:

- 2 cups edamame pods (fresh or frozen)
- 1 tablespoon olive oil
- 1-2 cloves garlic, minced

- 1 teaspoon sesame oil
- 1 tablespoon soy sauce
- 1 teaspoon sesame seeds (optional)
- 1/2 teaspoon red pepper flakes (optional)
- Salt to taste

Instructions:

1. If using frozen edamame, thaw them according to the package instructions.

2. In a pot of boiling water, add the edamame pods and cook for 3-5 minutes or until they are tender but still have a slight crunch.

3. Drain the edamame pods and transfer them to a bowl.

4. In a large skillet or wok, heat olive oil over medium-high heat.

5. Add minced garlic to the hot oil and sauté for about 30 seconds until fragrant.

6. Add the cooked edamame pods to the skillet and stir-fry for 2-3 minutes, ensuring they are well-coated in the garlic-infused oil.

7. Drizzle sesame oil and soy sauce over the edamame pods. Toss to combine.

8. If using, sprinkle sesame seeds and red pepper flakes over the edamame pods. Mix well.

9. Season with salt to taste.

10. Cook for an additional 2-3 minutes, stirring frequently, until the edamame pods are heated through and infused with flavors.

11. Transfer the edamame pods to a serving plate.

12. Serve immediately and enjoy this flavorful and nutritious snack.

Yogurt Parfait with Granola

Ingredients:

- 1 cup Greek yogurt
- 1/2 cup granola (store-bought or homemade)
- 1/2 cup mixed berries (strawberries, blueberries, raspberries)
- 1 tablespoon honey or maple syrup (optional)
- 1 tablespoon chia seeds (optional)
- 2 tablespoons chopped nuts (almonds, walnuts, or your choice)
- Fresh mint leaves for garnish (optional)

Instructions:

1. In a glass or serving bowl, spoon a layer of Greek yogurt to create the base.

2. Add a layer of granola on top of the yogurt.

3. Arrange a layer of mixed berries over the granola.

4. Optionally, drizzle honey or maple syrup over the berries for added sweetness.

5. Sprinkle chia seeds over the berries for an extra nutritional boost.

6. Repeat the layers until you reach the top of the glass or bowl, finishing with a final layer of mixed berries.

7. Garnish the Yogurt Parfait with chopped nuts and fresh mint leaves if desired.

8. Serve immediately and enjoy this delicious and nutritious yogurt parfait with granola.

Chia Seed Pudding Cups

Ingredients:

- 1/4 cup chia seeds
- 1 cup milk (dairy or plant-based)
- 1 tablespoon maple syrup or honey
- 1/2 teaspoon vanilla extract
- Fresh fruit (berries, mango, kiwi) for topping
- Nuts or seeds (almonds, walnuts, pumpkin seeds) for topping

- Optional: a pinch of cinnamon or a drizzle of nut butter for added flavor

Instructions:

1. In a bowl, combine chia seeds, milk, maple syrup (or honey), and vanilla extract. Whisk the ingredients together thoroughly.
2. Let the mixture sit for about 5 minutes, and then whisk again to prevent clumps.
3. Cover the bowl and refrigerate for at least 2 hours or preferably overnight to allow the chia seeds to absorb the liquid and create a pudding-like consistency.
4. Before serving, give the chia seed pudding a good stir to ensure an even texture.
5. Spoon the chia seed pudding into individual cups or jars.
6. Top each pudding cup with fresh fruit and nuts or seeds of your choice.
7. Optionally, sprinkle a pinch of cinnamon or drizzle nut butter over the toppings for added flavor.
8. Serve the Chia Seed Pudding Cups chilled and enjoy this nutritious and satisfying treat.

Apple Slices with Nut Butter

Ingredients:

- 2 apples (any variety), cored and sliced
- 1/4 cup almond butter, peanut butter, or your favorite nut butter
- 1 tablespoon honey or maple syrup (optional)
- 1 tablespoon chia seeds or flaxseeds (optional)
- 1 tablespoon chopped nuts (walnuts, almonds) for garnish
- Cinnamon for sprinkling (optional)
- Lemon juice (to prevent browning of apple slices)

Instructions:

1. Core and slice the apples. If not serving immediately, toss the apple slices with a bit of lemon juice to prevent browning.
2. In a small bowl, warm the nut butter in the microwave for about 15 seconds to make it easier to drizzle.
3. Arrange the apple slices on a serving plate.
4. Drizzle the nut butter over the apple slices.
5. Optionally, drizzle honey or maple syrup over the nut butter for added sweetness.

6. Sprinkle chia seeds or flaxseeds over the apple slices for an extra nutritional boost.

7. Garnish with chopped nuts and a sprinkle of cinnamon if desired.

8. Serve the Apple Slices with Nut Butter immediately and enjoy this simple, healthy, and satisfying snack.

Vegetable Chips with Guacamole

Ingredients:

For Vegetable Chips:

- 2 large sweet potatoes, thinly sliced
- 2 zucchinis, thinly sliced
- 1 large beet, thinly sliced
- 2 tablespoons olive oil
- 1 teaspoon paprika
- 1/2 teaspoon garlic powder
- Salt and pepper to taste

For Guacamole:

- 3 ripe avocados, peeled and pitted
- 1 tomato, diced
- 1/4 cup red onion, finely chopped
- 1/4 cup fresh cilantro, chopped
- 1 clove garlic, minced

- Juice of 1 lime
- Salt and pepper to taste

Instructions:

For Vegetable Chips:

1. Preheat the oven to 375°F (190°C). Line baking sheets with parchment paper.

2. In a large bowl, toss the sweet potato, zucchini, and beet slices with olive oil, paprika, garlic powder, salt, and pepper until well coated.

3. Arrange the vegetable slices in a single layer on the prepared baking sheets.

4. Bake in the preheated oven for 20-25 minutes or until the edges are crispy and golden brown. Flip the slices halfway through the baking time for even crispiness.

5. Remove from the oven and let the vegetable chips cool on the baking sheets.

For Guacamole:

1. In a bowl, mash the ripe avocados with a fork.

2. Add diced tomato, finely chopped red onion, chopped cilantro, minced garlic, lime juice, salt, and pepper to the mashed avocados.

3. Mix all the ingredients together until well combined.

4. Taste and adjust the seasoning as needed.

To Serve:

1. Arrange the vegetable chips on a serving platter.

2. Serve the Guacamole in a bowl alongside the vegetable chips.

3. Enjoy Vegetable Chips with Guacamole as a tasty and wholesome snack or appetizer.

Hard-Boiled Eggs with Cherry Tomatoes

Ingredients:

- 4 large eggs
- 1 cup cherry tomatoes, halved
- 1 tablespoon olive oil
- 1 teaspoon balsamic vinegar
- Salt and pepper to taste
- Fresh basil leaves for garnish (optional)

Instructions:

1. Place the eggs in a single layer in a saucepan and cover them with water.

2. Bring the water to a boil over medium-high heat.

3. Once boiling, reduce the heat to low, cover, and simmer for 9-12 minutes, depending on your desired yolk consistency (9 minutes for a creamy yolk, 12 minutes for a fully set yolk).

4. While the eggs are cooking, prepare an ice bath in a bowl or basin.

5. Once the eggs are done, transfer them immediately to the ice bath to cool for about 5 minutes.

6. Once cooled, peel the hard-boiled eggs and cut them in half lengthwise.

7. In a bowl, combine the halved cherry tomatoes with olive oil, balsamic vinegar, salt, and pepper. Toss gently to coat the tomatoes.

8. Arrange the hard-boiled egg halves on a serving plate.

9. Spoon the dressed cherry tomatoes over the eggs.

10. Optionally, garnish with fresh basil leaves for added freshness.

11. Serve the Hard-Boiled Eggs with Cherry Tomatoes as a light and nutritious snack or appetizer.

Roasted Chickpeas

Ingredients:

- 2 cans (15 oz each) chickpeas, drained and rinsed (or 3 cups cooked chickpeas)
- 2 tablespoons olive oil
- 1 teaspoon ground cumin
- 1 teaspoon smoked paprika
- 1/2 teaspoon garlic powder
- 1/2 teaspoon onion powder
- 1/4 teaspoon cayenne pepper (adjust to taste for spice)
- Salt to taste

Instructions:

1. Preheat the oven to 400°F (200°C). Line a baking sheet with parchment paper.
2. Rinse and drain the chickpeas. Pat them dry with a clean kitchen towel to remove excess moisture.
3. In a bowl, toss the chickpeas with olive oil, ground cumin, smoked paprika, garlic powder, onion powder, cayenne pepper, and salt. Ensure the chickpeas are well coated with the seasonings.
4. Spread the seasoned chickpeas in a single layer on the prepared baking sheet.

5. Roast in the preheated oven for 25-30 minutes or until the chickpeas are golden and crispy, shaking the pan occasionally for even cooking.

6. Remove from the oven and let the roasted chickpeas cool slightly before serving.

7. Optionally, sprinkle additional salt or your favorite spices over the chickpeas for extra flavor.

8. Serve the Roasted Chickpeas as a crunchy and protein-packed snack or use them as a topping for salads and soups.

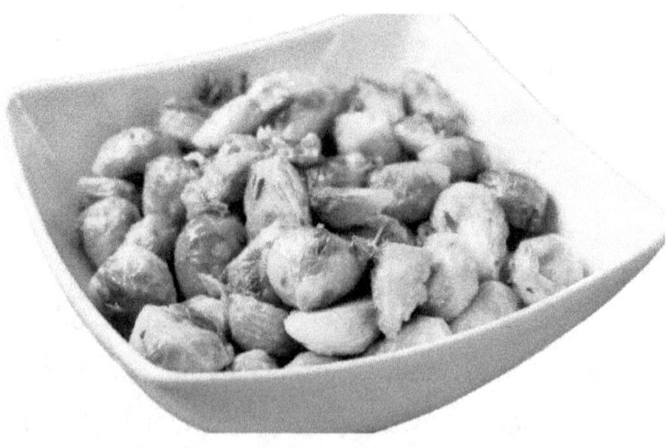

CHAPTER 7: VEGETABLE RECIPES

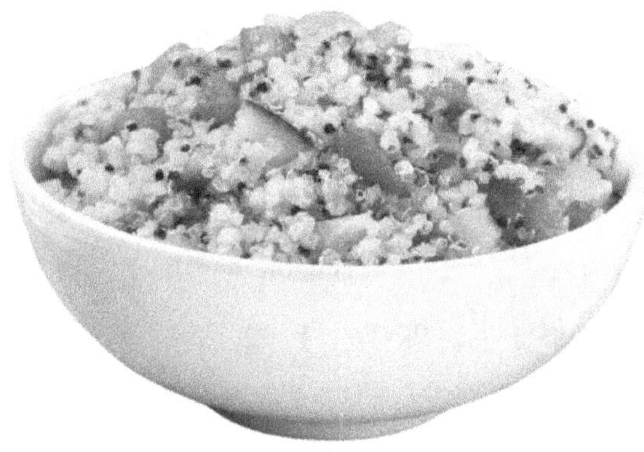

Roasted Brussels Sprouts and Sweet Potatoes

Ingredients:

- 1 lb Brussels sprouts, trimmed and halved
- 2 medium sweet potatoes, peeled and cut into 1-inch cubes
- 3 tablespoons olive oil
- 1 teaspoon garlic powder
- 1 teaspoon smoked paprika
- Salt and black pepper, to taste

- 2 tablespoons balsamic glaze (optional, for drizzling)

Instructions:

1. Preheat your oven to 425°F (220°C).

2. In a large mixing bowl, combine the Brussels sprouts and sweet potatoes.

3. Drizzle olive oil over the vegetables and toss to coat evenly.

4. Sprinkle garlic powder, smoked paprika, salt, and black pepper over the vegetables. Toss again to ensure even seasoning.

5. Spread the Brussels sprouts and sweet potatoes in a single layer on a baking sheet.

6. Roast in the preheated oven for about 25-30 minutes or until the vegetables are golden brown and crispy on the edges. Remember to toss halfway through the roasting time for even cooking.

7. Once roasted, remove from the oven and drizzle with balsamic glaze if desired. Toss gently to combine.

8. Serve immediately as a flavorful and nutritious side dish.

Grilled Zucchini and Eggplant Skewers

Ingredients:

- 2 medium zucchinis, sliced into 1/2-inch rounds
- 1 large eggplant, cut into 1-inch cubes
- 1/4 cup olive oil
- 2 cloves garlic, minced
- 1 teaspoon dried oregano
- 1 teaspoon dried thyme
- Salt and black pepper, to taste
- Wooden skewers, soaked in water for 30 minutes

Instructions:

1. Preheat your grill to medium-high heat.
2. In a bowl, mix together olive oil, minced garlic, dried oregano, dried thyme, salt, and black pepper.
3. Thread the zucchini rounds and eggplant cubes onto the soaked wooden skewers, alternating between them.
4. Brush the skewers with the prepared olive oil mixture, coating them evenly.
5. Place the skewers on the preheated grill and cook for about 8-10 minutes, turning

occasionally, until the vegetables are tender and have grill marks.

6. Remove the skewers from the grill and place them on a serving platter.

7. Optionally, garnish with fresh herbs like parsley or basil.

8. Serve the grilled zucchini and eggplant skewers as a delicious and healthy side dish.

Spinach and Mushroom Stuffed Bell Peppers

Ingredients:

- 4 large bell peppers, halved and seeds removed
- 2 cups fresh spinach, chopped
- 1 cup mushrooms, finely chopped
- 1 cup cooked quinoa or rice
- 1 cup shredded mozzarella cheese
- 1/2 cup grated Parmesan cheese
- 2 cloves garlic, minced
- 1 teaspoon dried oregano
- 1 teaspoon dried basil
- Salt and black pepper, to taste
- Olive oil for drizzling

Instructions:

1. Preheat your oven to 375°F (190°C).

2. Place the halved bell peppers in a baking dish.

3. In a skillet over medium heat, sauté the mushrooms until they release their moisture and become golden brown. Add chopped spinach and minced garlic, cooking until the spinach wilts.

4. In a large mixing bowl, combine the cooked quinoa or rice, sautéed mushrooms and spinach, mozzarella cheese, Parmesan cheese, dried oregano, dried basil, salt, and black pepper. Mix well.

5. Spoon the stuffing mixture into each bell pepper half, pressing down gently.

6. Drizzle a bit of olive oil over the stuffed peppers.

7. Cover the baking dish with foil and bake in the preheated oven for 25-30 minutes or until the peppers are tender.

8. Remove the foil and bake for an additional 5-10 minutes, allowing the cheese to melt and develop a golden crust.

9. Serve the spinach and mushroom stuffed bell peppers warm.

Tomato and Basil Salad

Ingredients:

- 4 large ripe tomatoes, sliced
- 1 cup cherry tomatoes, halved
- 1 cup fresh mozzarella cheese, diced
- 1/2 cup fresh basil leaves, torn
- 3 tablespoons extra-virgin olive oil
- 2 tablespoons balsamic vinegar
- Salt and black pepper, to taste
- 1 teaspoon honey (optional, for sweetness)

Instructions:

1. Arrange the sliced tomatoes, halved cherry tomatoes, and diced mozzarella on a serving platter.
2. Scatter torn fresh basil leaves over the tomatoes and mozzarella.
3. In a small bowl, whisk together extra-virgin olive oil, balsamic vinegar, salt, black pepper, and honey if using. Adjust the seasoning to taste.
4. Drizzle the dressing over the tomato, mozzarella, and basil mixture.
5. Gently toss the salad to coat the ingredients evenly with the dressing.

6. Allow the salad to sit for a few minutes to let the flavors meld.

7. Serve the tomato and basil salad as a refreshing side dish or appetizer.

Sweet Potato and Chickpea Curry

Ingredients:

- 2 medium sweet potatoes, peeled and diced
- 1 can (15 oz) chickpeas, drained and rinsed
- 1 large onion, finely chopped
- 3 cloves garlic, minced
- 1 tablespoon ginger, grated
- 1 can (14 oz) diced tomatoes
- 1 can (14 oz) coconut milk
- 2 tablespoons curry powder
- 1 teaspoon ground cumin
- 1 teaspoon ground coriander
- 1/2 teaspoon turmeric
- 1/4 teaspoon cayenne pepper (adjust to taste)
- Salt and black pepper, to taste
- 2 tablespoons vegetable oil
- Fresh cilantro, chopped (for garnish)
- Cooked rice (for serving)

Instructions:

1. In a large pot or deep skillet, heat vegetable oil over medium heat.
2. Add chopped onion and cook until softened and translucent.
3. Stir in minced garlic and grated ginger, cooking for an additional minute until fragrant.
4. Add curry powder, ground cumin, ground coriander, turmeric, and cayenne pepper to the pot. Stir well to coat the onions with the spices.
5. Add diced sweet potatoes, chickpeas, diced tomatoes (with their juices), and coconut milk to the pot. Season with salt and black pepper. Stir to combine.
6. Bring the mixture to a boil, then reduce the heat to low, cover, and simmer for about 20-25 minutes or until the sweet potatoes are tender.
7. Check the seasoning and adjust if needed.
8. Serve the sweet potato and chickpea curry over cooked rice, garnished with chopped cilantro.

Cabbage and Carrot Slaw

Ingredients:

- 4 cups green cabbage, finely shredded
- 2 cups carrots, grated
- 1/2 cup red onion, thinly sliced
- 1/4 cup fresh parsley, chopped
- 1/2 cup mayonnaise
- 2 tablespoons Dijon mustard
- 2 tablespoons apple cider vinegar
- 1 tablespoon honey
- Salt and black pepper, to taste

Instructions:

1. In a large bowl, combine shredded cabbage, grated carrots, sliced red onion, and chopped fresh parsley.

2. In a separate bowl, whisk together mayonnaise, Dijon mustard, apple cider vinegar, honey, salt, and black pepper. Adjust the seasoning to taste.

3. Pour the dressing over the cabbage and carrot mixture.

4. Toss the ingredients together until the slaw is evenly coated with the dressing.

5. Allow the slaw to sit in the refrigerator for at least 30 minutes before serving to allow the flavors to meld.

6. Before serving, give the slaw a final toss and adjust the seasoning if necessary.

7. Serve the cabbage and carrot slaw as a refreshing side dish or as a topping for sandwiches and tacos.

Spaghetti Squash Primavera

Ingredients:

- 1 medium spaghetti squash
- 2 tablespoons olive oil
- 1 small red bell pepper, thinly sliced
- 1 small yellow bell pepper, thinly sliced
- 1 medium zucchini, julienned
- 1 medium carrot, julienned
- 1 cup cherry tomatoes, halved
- 3 cloves garlic, minced
- 1/2 cup grated Parmesan cheese
- 1/4 cup fresh basil, chopped
- Salt and black pepper, to taste
- Crushed red pepper flakes (optional, for heat)

Instructions:

1. Preheat the oven to 375°F (190°C).

2. Cut the spaghetti squash in half lengthwise and scoop out the seeds. Place the squash halves, cut side down, on a baking sheet. Bake in the preheated oven for 40-50 minutes or until the squash is tender and the strands easily separate.

3. While the squash is baking, heat olive oil in a large skillet over medium heat.

4. Add minced garlic and sauté for about 1 minute until fragrant.

5. Add sliced red and yellow bell peppers, julienned zucchini, and julienned carrot to the skillet. Cook for 5-7 minutes, or until the vegetables are tender-crisp.

6. Stir in cherry tomatoes and cook for an additional 2-3 minutes until they start to soften.

7. Once the spaghetti squash is done, use a fork to scrape the flesh into spaghetti-like strands.

8. Add the spaghetti squash to the skillet with the sautéed vegetables. Toss everything together until well combined.

9. Season the dish with salt, black pepper, and crushed red pepper flakes if desired.

10. Sprinkle grated Parmesan cheese and chopped fresh basil over the top.

11. Toss once more and cook for an additional 2-3 minutes until everything is heated through.

12. Serve the spaghetti squash primavera warm, garnished with extra Parmesan and basil if desired.

Baked Salmon with Asparagus

Ingredients:

- 4 salmon filets
- 1 bunch asparagus, tough ends trimmed
- 2 tablespoons olive oil
- 2 tablespoons fresh lemon juice
- 3 cloves garlic, minced
- 1 teaspoon dried oregano
- Salt and black pepper, to taste
- Lemon slices (for garnish)
- Fresh parsley, chopped (for garnish)

Instructions:

1. Preheat your oven to 400°F (200°C).

2. Place the salmon filets on a baking sheet lined with parchment paper.

3. Arrange the trimmed asparagus around the salmon on the baking sheet.

4. In a small bowl, whisk together olive oil, fresh lemon juice, minced garlic, dried oregano, salt, and black pepper.

5. Drizzle half of the prepared olive oil mixture over the salmon filets, ensuring they are well-coated.

6. Drizzle the remaining half of the mixture over the asparagus.

7. Season the salmon filets with additional salt and pepper if desired.

8. Place lemon slices on top of the salmon filets for added flavor.

9. Bake in the preheated oven for about 12-15 minutes, or until the salmon is cooked through and flakes easily with a fork.

10. The asparagus should be tender but still slightly crisp.

11. Garnish with fresh chopped parsley before serving.

12. Serve the baked salmon with asparagus hot, and enjoy a healthy and flavorful meal.

Cauliflower Rice Stir-Fry

Ingredients:

- 1 medium-sized cauliflower, grated into rice-like texture
- 1 cup mixed vegetables (e.g., bell peppers, broccoli, carrots, peas)
- 1 cup firm tofu or cooked chicken, diced (optional)
- 3 tablespoons soy sauce
- 2 tablespoons sesame oil
- 1 tablespoon ginger, minced
- 2 cloves garlic, minced
- 1 tablespoon vegetable oil
- 2 green onions, sliced (for garnish)
- Sesame seeds (optional, for garnish)

Instructions:

1. Heat vegetable oil in a large skillet or wok over medium-high heat.
2. Add minced ginger and garlic to the hot oil, sautéing for about 1 minute until fragrant.
3. Add the grated cauliflower rice to the skillet and stir-fry for 5-7 minutes, or until it's cooked through and slightly crispy.

4. Push the cauliflower rice to the side of the skillet, and add a bit more oil if needed. If using tofu or chicken, cook it until browned and cooked through.

5. Add the mixed vegetables to the skillet and stir-fry for an additional 3-5 minutes, or until they are tender-crisp.

6. Pour soy sauce and sesame oil over the cauliflower rice and vegetables. Toss everything together until well combined.

7. If using tofu or chicken, make sure it's evenly distributed throughout the stir-fry.

8. Cook for an additional 2-3 minutes, allowing the flavors to meld.

9. Garnish with sliced green onions and sesame seeds, if desired.

10. Serve the cauliflower rice stir-fry hot, either as a side dish or a light main course.

Brussels Sprouts and Pomegranate Salad

Ingredients:

- 1 lb Brussels sprouts, trimmed and thinly sliced
- 1 cup pomegranate seeds

- 1/2 cup feta cheese, crumbled
- 1/2 cup walnuts, toasted and chopped
- 1/4 cup red onion, thinly sliced
- 2 tablespoons balsamic vinegar
- 3 tablespoons olive oil
- 1 tablespoon honey
- Salt and black pepper, to taste

Instructions:

1. In a large bowl, combine thinly sliced Brussels sprouts, pomegranate seeds, crumbled feta cheese, toasted and chopped walnuts, and thinly sliced red onion.

2. In a small bowl, whisk together balsamic vinegar, olive oil, honey, salt, and black pepper. Adjust the dressing to taste.

3. Pour the dressing over the Brussels sprouts and pomegranate mixture.

4. Toss the salad until all ingredients are evenly coated with the dressing.

5. Allow the salad to sit for a few minutes to let the flavors meld.

6. Before serving, give it a final toss and adjust the seasoning if necessary.

7. Serve the Brussels sprouts and pomegranate salad as a vibrant and flavorful side dish.

Garlic Lemon Shrimp with Broccoli

Ingredients:

- 1 lb large shrimp, peeled and deveined
- 3 cups broccoli florets
- 4 cloves garlic, minced
- Zest of 1 lemon
- Juice of 1 lemon
- 3 tablespoons olive oil
- 1/2 teaspoon red pepper flakes (optional, for heat)
- Salt and black pepper, to taste
- Fresh parsley, chopped (for garnish)

Instructions:

1. In a large skillet or pan, heat olive oil over medium-high heat.
2. Add minced garlic to the hot oil and sauté for about 1 minute until fragrant.
3. Add the shrimp to the skillet, cooking for 2-3 minutes on each side until they turn pink and opaque.

4. Remove the cooked shrimp from the skillet and set aside.

5. In the same skillet, add broccoli florets. Cook for 3-4 minutes, or until they are tender-crisp.

6. Return the cooked shrimp to the skillet with the broccoli.

7. Add lemon zest, lemon juice, red pepper flakes (if using), salt, and black pepper. Toss everything together until well combined.

8. Cook for an additional 2-3 minutes to allow the flavors to meld.

9. Garnish with chopped fresh parsley.

10. Serve the garlic lemon shrimp with broccoli hot, over rice or your preferred grain.

CHAPTER 8: SALAD RECIPES

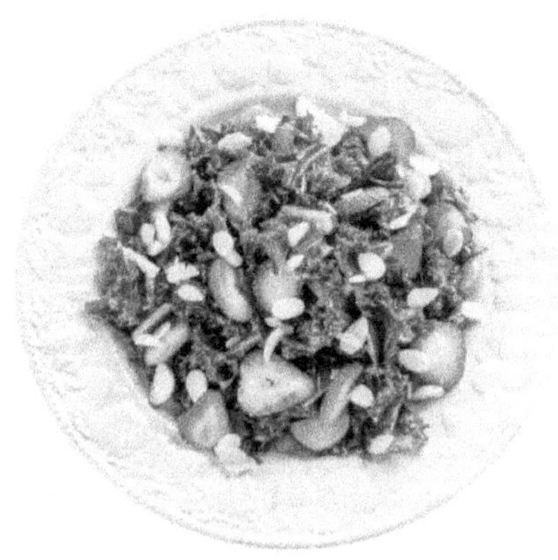

Kale and Berry Salad with Almonds

Ingredients:

For the Salad:

- 6 cups kale, stems removed and chopped
- 1 cup fresh blueberries
- 1 cup fresh strawberries, hulled and sliced
- 1/2 cup sliced almonds, toasted

For the Dressing:

- 1/4 cup olive oil
- 2 tablespoons balsamic vinegar
- 1 tablespoon honey
- 1 teaspoon Dijon mustard

- Salt and black pepper to taste

Instructions:

1. In a large salad bowl, place the chopped kale.
2. In a small skillet, toast the sliced almonds over medium heat until they become golden brown and fragrant. Keep an eye on them to prevent burning.
3. Add the toasted almonds, fresh blueberries, and sliced strawberries to the kale in the salad bowl.
4. In a separate small bowl, whisk together olive oil, balsamic vinegar, honey, Dijon mustard, salt, and black pepper. Adjust the sweetness and acidity to your liking.
5. Pour the dressing over the kale and berries. Toss the salad until the ingredients are well coated with the dressing.
6. Allow the salad to sit for a few minutes to let the kale absorb the flavors of the dressing.
7. Serve the Kale and Berry Salad with a sprinkle of additional almonds on top for added crunch.

Quinoa Salad with Roasted Vegetables

Ingredients:

For the Roasted Vegetables:

- 2 cups cherry tomatoes, halved
- 1 medium-sized zucchini, diced
- 1 red bell pepper, diced
- 1 yellow bell pepper, diced
- 1 red onion, sliced
- 3 tablespoons olive oil
- 1 teaspoon dried oregano
- Salt and black pepper to taste

For the Quinoa Salad:

- 1 cup quinoa, rinsed and drained
- 2 cups water or vegetable broth
- 1/4 cup olive oil
- 2 tablespoons balsamic vinegar
- 1 teaspoon Dijon mustard
- 1 clove garlic, minced
- Salt and black pepper to taste
- 1/2 cup crumbled feta cheese (optional)
- 1/4 cup chopped fresh parsley

Instructions:

For the Roasted Vegetables:

1. Preheat your oven to 400°F (200°C).

2. In a large bowl, combine halved cherry tomatoes, diced zucchini, diced red and yellow bell peppers, and sliced red onion.

3. Drizzle olive oil over the vegetables and sprinkle with dried oregano, salt, and black pepper. Toss until the vegetables are evenly coated.

4. Spread the vegetables on a baking sheet in a single layer.

5. Roast in the preheated oven for 25-30 minutes or until the vegetables are tender and slightly caramelized, stirring halfway through.

For the Quinoa Salad:

1. In a medium saucepan, combine quinoa and water or vegetable broth. Bring to a boil, then reduce heat to low, cover, and simmer for 15 minutes or until the quinoa is cooked and the liquid is absorbed.

2. In a small bowl, whisk together olive oil, balsamic vinegar, Dijon mustard, minced garlic, salt, and black pepper to create the dressing.

3. Fluff the cooked quinoa with a fork and transfer it to a large salad bowl.

4. Add the roasted vegetables to the quinoa.

5. Pour the dressing over the quinoa and vegetables. Toss everything together until well combined.

6. If using, sprinkle crumbled feta cheese and chopped fresh parsley over the quinoa salad.

7. Serve the Quinoa Salad with Roasted Vegetables at room temperature or chilled.

Citrus Avocado Salad with Shrimp

Ingredients:

For the Citrus Avocado Salad:

- 4 cups mixed salad greens (arugula, spinach, or your choice)
- 2 avocados, peeled, pitted, and sliced
- 1 grapefruit, peeled and segmented
- 2 oranges, peeled and segmented
- 1/2 red onion, thinly sliced
- 1/4 cup chopped fresh mint
- 1/4 cup crumbled feta cheese (optional)

For the Shrimp:

- 1 pound large shrimp, peeled and deveined
- 2 tablespoons olive oil
- 1 teaspoon smoked paprika
- 1 teaspoon ground cumin

- Salt and black pepper to taste
- Zest of 1 lemon

For the Citrus Vinaigrette:

- 1/4 cup olive oil
- 2 tablespoons fresh orange juice
- 2 tablespoons fresh lemon juice
- 1 tablespoon honey
- 1 teaspoon Dijon mustard
- Salt and black pepper to taste

Instructions:

For the Shrimp:

1. In a bowl, combine peeled and deveined shrimp with olive oil, smoked paprika, ground cumin, salt, black pepper, and lemon zest. Toss to coat the shrimp evenly.

2. Heat a skillet over medium-high heat. Add the seasoned shrimp and cook for 2-3 minutes per side or until they are opaque and cooked through. Set aside.

For the Citrus Avocado Salad:

1. In a large salad bowl, combine mixed salad greens, sliced avocados, grapefruit segments, orange segments, thinly sliced red onion, and chopped fresh mint. If using, sprinkle crumbled feta cheese over the salad.

For the Citrus Vinaigrette:

1. In a small bowl, whisk together olive oil, fresh orange juice, fresh lemon juice, honey, Dijon mustard, salt, and black pepper.
2. Drizzle the citrus vinaigrette over the salad and toss gently to combine.

To Assemble:

1. Arrange the cooked shrimp on top of the Citrus Avocado Salad.
2. Serve immediately, and enjoy this Citrus Avocado Salad with Shrimp as a refreshing and flavorful meal.

Chickpea and Cucumber Salad

Ingredients:

- 2 cans (15 ounces each) chickpeas, drained and rinsed
- 1 cucumber, diced
- 1 cup cherry tomatoes, halved
- 1/2 red onion, finely chopped
- 1/4 cup fresh parsley, chopped
- 1/4 cup feta cheese, crumbled (optional)

For the Dressing:

- 3 tablespoons olive oil

- 2 tablespoons red wine vinegar
- 1 teaspoon Dijon mustard
- 1 clove garlic, minced
- Salt and black pepper to taste

Instructions:

1. In a large salad bowl, combine chickpeas, diced cucumber, halved cherry tomatoes, finely chopped red onion, and chopped fresh parsley.
2. If using, add crumbled feta cheese to the salad.

For the Dressing:

1. In a small bowl, whisk together olive oil, red wine vinegar, Dijon mustard, minced garlic, salt, and black pepper until well combined.
2. Pour the dressing over the chickpea and cucumber mixture.
3. Toss the salad gently to ensure all ingredients are coated with the dressing.
4. Allow the salad to marinate in the refrigerator for at least 30 minutes to let the flavors meld.
5. Before serving, give the salad a final toss and adjust the seasoning if necessary.
6. Serve the Chickpea and Cucumber Salad as a refreshing side dish or a light meal.

Grilled Chicken Caesar Salad with Whole Grain Croutons

Ingredients:

For Grilled Chicken:

- 4 boneless, skinless chicken breasts
- 2 tablespoons olive oil
- 1 teaspoon garlic powder
- 1 teaspoon dried oregano
- Salt and black pepper to taste
- Juice of 1 lemon

For Whole Grain Croutons:

- 4 cups whole grain bread, cubed
- 2 tablespoons olive oil
- 1 teaspoon garlic powder
- 1 teaspoon dried thyme
- Salt and black pepper to taste

For Caesar Salad:

- 2 heads romaine lettuce, chopped
- 1 cup cherry tomatoes, halved
- 1/2 cup shaved Parmesan cheese
- Caesar dressing (store-bought or homemade)

Instructions:

For Grilled Chicken:

1. In a bowl, mix olive oil, garlic powder, dried oregano, salt, black pepper, and lemon juice to create a marinade.

2. Place chicken breasts in a zip-top bag or shallow dish and pour the marinade over them. Ensure the chicken is well coated. Marinate in the refrigerator for at least 30 minutes.

3. Preheat the grill to medium-high heat. Grill the chicken for about 6-8 minutes per side or until cooked through. Let it rest for a few minutes before slicing.

For Whole Grain Croutons:

1. Preheat your oven to 375°F (190°C).

2. In a bowl, toss cubed whole grain bread with olive oil, garlic powder, dried thyme, salt, and black pepper until the bread is evenly coated.

3. Spread the seasoned bread cubes on a baking sheet in a single layer.

4. Bake in the preheated oven for 12-15 minutes or until the croutons are golden and crispy. Stir them halfway through the baking time.

For Caesar Salad:

1. In a large salad bowl, combine chopped romaine lettuce, halved cherry tomatoes, and shaved Parmesan cheese.

2. Add the grilled chicken slices on top.

3. Sprinkle whole grain croutons over the salad.

4. Drizzle Caesar dressing over the salad or serve it on the side.

5. Toss the salad just before serving to coat the ingredients with the dressing.

Mango and Black Bean Salad

Ingredients:

- 2 ripe mangoes, peeled, pitted, and diced
- 1 can (15 ounces) black beans, drained and rinsed
- 1 red bell pepper, diced
- 1/2 red onion, finely chopped
- 1 cup corn kernels (fresh, frozen, or canned)
- 1/4 cup fresh cilantro, chopped
- Juice of 2 limes
- 3 tablespoons olive oil
- 1 teaspoon ground cumin
- 1/2 teaspoon chili powder

- Salt and black pepper to taste
- Optional: Avocado slices for garnish

Instructions:

1. In a large salad bowl, combine diced mangoes, black beans, diced red bell pepper, finely chopped red onion, corn kernels, and chopped fresh cilantro.

2. In a small bowl, whisk together lime juice, olive oil, ground cumin, chili powder, salt, and black pepper to create the dressing.

3. Pour the dressing over the mango and black bean mixture.

4. Toss the salad gently to ensure all ingredients are well coated with the dressing.

5. Adjust salt and pepper to taste.

6. If desired, garnish the salad with slices of ripe avocado.

7. Allow the salad to chill in the refrigerator for at least 30 minutes before serving to let the flavors meld.

8. Serve the Mango and Black Bean Salad as a refreshing side dish or a light and nutritious meal.

Arugula and Watermelon Salad

Ingredients:

- 4 cups arugula, washed and dried
- 3 cups seedless watermelon, cubed
- 1/2 cup crumbled feta cheese
- 1/4 cup fresh mint leaves, chopped
- 1/4 cup red onion, thinly sliced
- 1/2 cup chopped cucumber
- 1/4 cup extra virgin olive oil
- 2 tablespoons balsamic vinegar
- Salt and black pepper to taste

Instructions:

1. In a large salad bowl, combine arugula, cubed watermelon, crumbled feta cheese, chopped fresh mint, thinly sliced red onion, and chopped cucumber.
2. In a small bowl, whisk together extra virgin olive oil, balsamic vinegar, salt, and black pepper to create the dressing.
3. Drizzle the dressing over the salad ingredients.
4. Toss the salad gently to ensure all ingredients are well coated with the dressing.
5. Adjust salt and pepper to taste.

6. Allow the salad to chill in the refrigerator for about 15-20 minutes before serving.

7. Serve the Arugula and Watermelon Salad as a refreshing side dish or a light and hydrating summer salad.

Broccoli Salad with Cranberries and Sunflower Seeds

Ingredients:

For the Salad:

- 4 cups fresh broccoli florets, blanched and cooled
- 1/2 cup red onion, finely chopped
- 1/2 cup dried cranberries
- 1/2 cup sunflower seeds, toasted
- 1/2 cup crispy bacon, crumbled (optional)

For the Dressing:

- 1 cup mayonnaise
- 1/4 cup apple cider vinegar
- 1/4 cup honey
- 1 tablespoon Dijon mustard
- Salt and black pepper to taste

Instructions:

1. Blanch the broccoli florets in boiling water for about 1-2 minutes, then immediately transfer them to an ice water bath to stop the cooking process. Drain and pat them dry with a clean kitchen towel.

2. In a large salad bowl, combine blanched broccoli florets, finely chopped red onion, dried cranberries, toasted sunflower seeds, and crispy bacon (if using).

3. In a separate bowl, whisk together mayonnaise, apple cider vinegar, honey, Dijon mustard, salt, and black pepper to create the dressing.

4. Pour the dressing over the broccoli mixture.

5. Toss the salad gently to ensure all ingredients are well coated with the dressing.

6. Adjust salt and pepper to taste.

7. Allow the Broccoli Salad with Cranberries and Sunflower Seeds to chill in the refrigerator for at least 30 minutes before serving.

8. Serve the salad as a delicious and crunchy side dish.

Tuna and White Bean Salad

Ingredients:

- 2 cans (15 ounces each) white beans, drained and rinsed
- 2 cans (5 ounces each) tuna, drained
- 1/2 red onion, finely chopped
- 1/2 cup cherry tomatoes, halved
- 1/4 cup Kalamata olives, sliced
- 1/4 cup fresh parsley, chopped
- 2 tablespoons capers, drained
- 1/4 cup extra virgin olive oil
- 2 tablespoons red wine vinegar
- 1 teaspoon Dijon mustard
- Salt and black pepper to taste
- Optional: Feta cheese crumbles for garnish

Instructions:

1. In a large salad bowl, combine white beans, drained tuna, finely chopped red onion, halved cherry tomatoes, sliced Kalamata olives, chopped fresh parsley, and capers.

2. In a small bowl, whisk together extra virgin olive oil, red wine vinegar, Dijon mustard, salt, and black pepper to create the dressing.

3. Pour the dressing over the tuna and white bean mixture.

4. Toss the salad gently to ensure all ingredients are well coated with the dressing.

5. Adjust salt and pepper to taste.

6. If desired, sprinkle feta cheese crumbles over the salad for added flavor.

7. Allow the Tuna and White Bean Salad to chill in the refrigerator for at least 30 minutes before serving.

8. Serve the salad as a protein-packed and flavorful meal.

Asian-Inspired Quinoa Salad

Ingredients:

For the Quinoa Salad:

- 1 cup quinoa, rinsed and drained
- 2 cups water or vegetable broth
- 1 red bell pepper, thinly sliced
- 1 carrot, julienned
- 1 cup shredded purple cabbage
- 1 cup edamame, cooked and shelled
- 1/4 cup green onions, thinly sliced
- 1/4 cup cilantro, chopped

- 1/4 cup roasted peanuts, chopped (optional)
- Sesame seeds for garnish (optional)

For the Dressing:

- 3 tablespoons soy sauce
- 2 tablespoons rice vinegar
- 1 tablespoon sesame oil
- 1 tablespoon honey or maple syrup
- 1 clove garlic, minced
- 1 teaspoon fresh ginger, grated
- 1 tablespoon lime juice
- 1 teaspoon Sriracha sauce (adjust to taste)

Instructions:

For the Quinoa Salad:

1. In a medium saucepan, combine quinoa and water or vegetable broth. Bring to a boil, then reduce heat to low, cover, and simmer for 15 minutes or until the quinoa is cooked and the liquid is absorbed.
2. Fluff the quinoa with a fork and let it cool to room temperature.
3. In a large salad bowl, combine cooked quinoa, thinly sliced red bell pepper, julienned carrot, shredded purple cabbage, cooked edamame, sliced green onions, chopped cilantro, and chopped roasted peanuts (if using).

For the Dressing:

1. In a small bowl, whisk together soy sauce, rice vinegar, sesame oil, honey or maple syrup, minced garlic, grated ginger, lime juice, and Sriracha sauce.
2. Pour the dressing over the quinoa and vegetable mixture.
3. Toss the salad gently to ensure all ingredients are well coated with the dressing.
4. Adjust Sriracha sauce or honey/maple syrup to achieve the desired balance of sweet and spicy.
5. Garnish the salad with sesame seeds, if desired.
6. Allow the Asian-Inspired Quinoa Salad to chill in the refrigerator for at least 30 minutes before serving.
7. Serve the salad as a refreshing and nutritious meal.

Pomegranate and Walnut Spinach Salad

Ingredients:

For the Salad:

- 6 cups baby spinach, washed and dried
- 1 cup pomegranate arils

- 1 cup walnuts, toasted and chopped
- 1/2 cup crumbled feta cheese (optional)
- 1/4 cup red onion, thinly sliced

For the Pomegranate Vinaigrette:

- 1/4 cup pomegranate juice
- 3 tablespoons extra virgin olive oil
- 1 tablespoon red wine vinegar
- 1 tablespoon honey
- 1 teaspoon Dijon mustard
- Salt and black pepper to taste

Instructions:

For the Salad:

1. In a large salad bowl, combine baby spinach, pomegranate arils, toasted and chopped walnuts, crumbled feta cheese (if using), and thinly sliced red onion.

For the Pomegranate Vinaigrette:

1. In a small bowl, whisk together pomegranate juice, extra virgin olive oil, red wine vinegar, honey, Dijon mustard, salt, and black pepper.
2. Drizzle the pomegranate vinaigrette over the salad ingredients.
3. Toss the salad gently to ensure all ingredients are well coated with the dressing.

4. Adjust salt and pepper to taste.

5. Allow the Pomegranate and Walnut Spinach Salad to chill in the refrigerator for about 15-20 minutes before serving.

6. Serve the salad as a refreshing and vibrant side dish or a light meal.

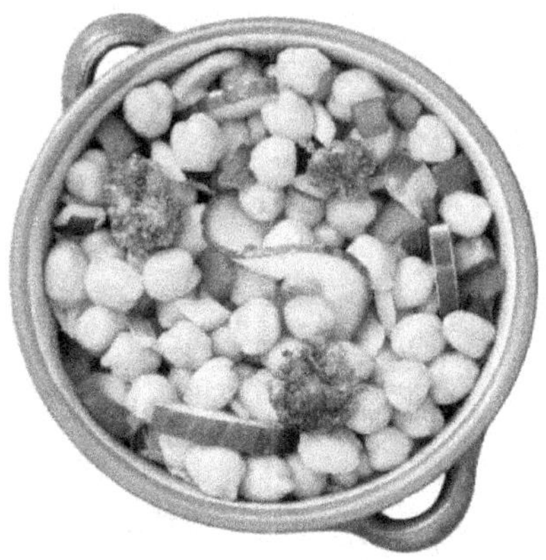

"I embrace the healing

power of gratitude in my

life."

"I am not defined by my

illness; I am defined by my

strength and resilience."

CHAPTER 9: DESSERT RECIPES

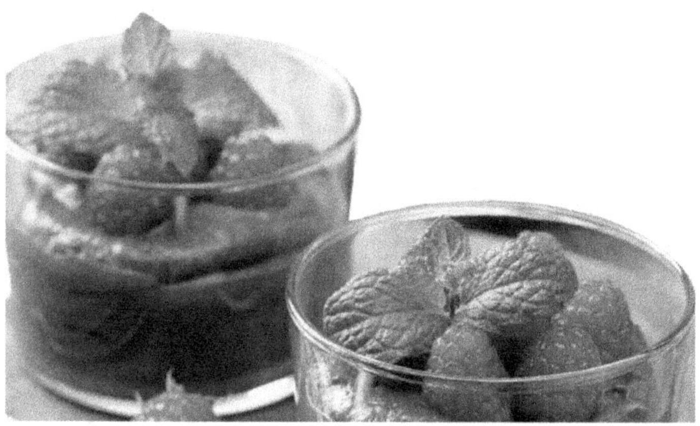

Berry and Yogurt Parfait

Ingredients:

- 2 cups mixed berries (strawberries, blueberries, raspberries)
- 2 cups Greek yogurt (vanilla or plain)
- 1 cup granola
- 2 tablespoons honey
- 1/4 cup sliced almonds (optional)

Instructions:

1. Wash and prepare the berries. If using strawberries, hull and slice them.
2. In serving glasses or bowls, begin by layering a spoonful of Greek yogurt at the bottom.

3. Add a layer of mixed berries on top of the yogurt.

4. Sprinkle a layer of granola over the berries.

5. Drizzle a little honey over the granola layer.

6. Repeat the layers until you reach the top of the glass or bowl, finishing with a final drizzle of honey.

7. If desired, top the parfait with sliced almonds for added crunch.

8. Repeat the layering process for additional parfaits.

9. Serve the Berry and Yogurt Parfait immediately, or refrigerate until ready to serve.

10. Enjoy this delightful and nutritious parfait as a breakfast or a healthy dessert option.

Baked Apples with Cinnamon and Walnuts

Ingredients:

- 4 medium-sized apples (such as Honeycrisp or Granny Smith)
- 1/4 cup chopped walnuts
- 2 tablespoons brown sugar
- 1 teaspoon ground cinnamon

- 2 tablespoons unsalted butter, melted
- 1/2 cup apple juice or cider
- Vanilla ice cream or whipped cream for serving (optional)

Instructions:

1. Preheat your oven to 375°F (190°C).
2. Wash the apples, and core them using an apple corer or a knife, leaving the bottom intact to create a well for the filling.
3. In a small bowl, mix together chopped walnuts, brown sugar, ground cinnamon, and melted butter to create the filling.
4. Place the cored apples in a baking dish, standing upright.
5. Stuff each apple with the walnut and cinnamon filling, pressing it down gently.
6. Pour apple juice or cider into the bottom of the baking dish to prevent the apples from drying out during baking.
7. Bake in the preheated oven for 25-30 minutes or until the apples are tender but not mushy.
8. Remove the baked apples from the oven and let them cool slightly before serving.

9. Optionally, serve the Baked Apples with a scoop of vanilla ice cream or a dollop of whipped cream.

10. Enjoy this warm and comforting dessert with the delightful flavors of cinnamon, walnuts, and baked apples.

Chocolate Avocado Mousse

Ingredients:

- 2 ripe avocados, peeled and pitted
- 1/2 cup cocoa powder
- 1/2 cup maple syrup or honey
- 1/4 cup almond milk or any milk of your choice
- 1 teaspoon vanilla extract
- A pinch of salt
- Optional toppings: whipped cream, berries, or shaved chocolate

Instructions:

1. Scoop the flesh of the ripe avocados into a blender or food processor.

2. Add cocoa powder, maple syrup or honey, almond milk, vanilla extract, and a pinch of salt to the blender.

3. Blend the ingredients until smooth and creamy. Stop and scrape down the sides of the blender or food processor if needed.

4. Taste the mixture and adjust the sweetness if necessary by adding more maple syrup or honey.

5. Once the mixture is smooth and well combined, transfer the chocolate avocado mousse to serving glasses or bowls.

6. Refrigerate the mousse for at least 30 minutes to allow it to chill and firm up.

7. Before serving, add optional toppings such as a dollop of whipped cream, fresh berries, or shaved chocolate.

8. Serve the Chocolate Avocado Mousse chilled and enjoy the rich and creamy chocolate flavor with the added benefit of avocado's natural creaminess.

Frozen Banana Bites

Ingredients:

- 3 ripe bananas
- 1/2 cup peanut butter or almond butter
- 1 cup dark chocolate chips or melting chocolate
- 1 tablespoon coconut oil (optional)

- Toppings of your choice (chopped nuts, shredded coconut, sprinkles)

Instructions:

1. Peel the bananas and cut them into bite-sized rounds, about 1/2 inch thick.

2. Spread a small amount of peanut butter or almond butter on half of the banana rounds.

3. Create banana sandwiches by placing the remaining banana rounds on top of the ones spread with nut butter, forming little banana bites.

4. Place the banana bites on a parchment paper-lined tray and freeze them for at least 1-2 hours until they are firm.

5. In a microwave-safe bowl or using a double boiler, melt the dark chocolate chips with coconut oil (if using) until smooth and well combined. Stir the mixture to ensure a silky consistency.

6. Remove the frozen banana bites from the freezer.

7. Using a fork, dip each banana bite into the melted chocolate, ensuring it is completely coated. Allow any excess chocolate to drip off.

8. Place the chocolate-covered banana bites back on the parchment paper-lined tray.

9. Sprinkle your favorite toppings over the chocolate while it's still wet, such as chopped nuts, shredded coconut, or sprinkles.

10. Return the tray to the freezer and let the frozen banana bites set for at least 1-2 hours or until the chocolate is fully hardened.

11. Once frozen, transfer the banana bites to an airtight container and store them in the freezer.

12. Serve the Frozen Banana Bites straight from the freezer and enjoy this delicious and healthier frozen treat.

Chia Seed Pudding with Fresh Fruit

Ingredients:

- 1/4 cup chia seeds
- 1 cup almond milk or any milk of your choice
- 1-2 tablespoons honey or maple syrup (adjust to taste)
- 1/2 teaspoon vanilla extract
- Fresh fruits for topping (berries, sliced kiwi, mango, etc.)

Instructions:

1. In a bowl, combine chia seeds, almond milk, honey or maple syrup, and vanilla extract.

2. Whisk the mixture well to ensure the chia seeds are evenly distributed.

3. Let the mixture sit for about 5 minutes, then whisk again to prevent clumping.

4. Cover the bowl and refrigerate the chia seed mixture for at least 3 hours or overnight to allow it to thicken.

5. Stir the chia seed pudding before serving to achieve a smooth and consistent texture.

6. Spoon the chia seed pudding into serving bowls or glasses.

7. Top the pudding with fresh fruits of your choice, such as berries, sliced kiwi, or mango.

8. Drizzle a little extra honey or maple syrup on top if desired.

9. Serve the Chia Seed Pudding with Fresh Fruit chilled and enjoy this nutritious and delicious breakfast or snack.

Mixed Berry Sorbet

Ingredients:

- 3 cups mixed berries (strawberries, blueberries, raspberries, blackberries)
- 1/2 cup granulated sugar
- 1 tablespoon lemon juice
- 1/2 cup water

Instructions:

1. Wash the berries thoroughly and remove any stems.
2. In a small saucepan, combine sugar and water over medium heat. Stir until the sugar is completely dissolved to create a simple syrup. Let it cool.
3. In a blender or food processor, combine the mixed berries and lemon juice.
4. Pour the cooled simple syrup over the berries in the blender.
5. Blend the mixture until smooth.
6. Strain the berry mixture through a fine-mesh sieve or cheesecloth to remove seeds and pulp, if desired. This step is optional, depending on your preference for a smoother sorbet.

7. Transfer the strained mixture to an ice cream maker and churn according to the manufacturer's instructions until it reaches a sorbet consistency.

8. If you don't have an ice cream maker, you can pour the mixture into a shallow dish and place it in the freezer. Every 30 minutes, stir the mixture with a fork to break up any ice crystals until it reaches a sorbet consistency (usually about 2-3 hours).

9. Once the sorbet reaches the desired consistency, transfer it to an airtight container and freeze for an additional hour to firm up.

10. Serve the Mixed Berry Sorbet in bowls or cones and enjoy this refreshing and fruity frozen treat!

Coconut and Almond Energy Balls

Ingredients:
- 1 cup rolled oats
- 1/2 cup shredded coconut (unsweetened)
- 1/2 cup almond butter
- 1/3 cup honey or maple syrup
- 1/2 cup ground almonds
- 1/4 cup chia seeds
- 1 teaspoon vanilla extract

- A pinch of salt

- Additional shredded coconut for rolling (optional)

Instructions:

1. In a large mixing bowl, combine rolled oats, shredded coconut, almond butter, honey or maple syrup, ground almonds, chia seeds, vanilla extract, and a pinch of salt.

2. Mix the ingredients thoroughly until well combined. If the mixture is too dry, you can add a little more almond butter or honey to achieve the desired consistency.

3. Place the mixture in the refrigerator for about 15-30 minutes to make it easier to handle.

4. After chilling, take small portions of the mixture and roll them into bite-sized balls using your hands.

5. If desired, roll the energy balls in additional shredded coconut to coat the exterior.

6. Place the coconut and almond energy balls on a parchment paper-lined tray or plate.

7. Refrigerate the energy balls for at least 1-2 hours to allow them to firm up.

8. Once chilled, transfer the energy balls to an airtight container and store them in the refrigerator.

9. Enjoy the Coconut and Almond Energy Balls as a quick and nutritious snack.

Orange and Pistachio Quinoa Cake

Ingredients:

For the Quinoa Cake:

- 1 cup quinoa, rinsed
- 2 cups water
- 1/2 cup unsalted butter, melted and cooled
- 3 large eggs
- 1 cup granulated sugar
- 1 cup plain Greek yogurt
- 1 teaspoon vanilla extract
- Zest of 2 oranges
- 1 1/2 cups all-purpose flour
- 2 teaspoons baking powder
- 1/2 teaspoon baking soda
- 1/4 teaspoon salt
- 1/2 cup shelled pistachios, chopped

For the Orange Glaze:

- 1 cup powdered sugar

- 2 tablespoons fresh orange juice
- Zest of 1 orange
- Chopped pistachios for garnish (optional)

Instructions:

For the Quinoa Cake:

1. In a medium saucepan, combine quinoa and water. Bring to a boil, then reduce heat to low, cover, and simmer for 15 minutes or until the quinoa is cooked and the water is absorbed. Let it cool.

2. Preheat your oven to 350°F (175°C). Grease and flour a 9-inch round cake pan.

3. In a large mixing bowl, whisk together melted butter, eggs, granulated sugar, Greek yogurt, vanilla extract, and orange zest.

4. In a separate bowl, combine the cooked quinoa, all-purpose flour, baking powder, baking soda, and salt. Gradually add the dry ingredients to the wet ingredients, mixing until well combined.

5. Fold in the chopped pistachios.

6. Pour the batter into the prepared cake pan and smooth the top with a spatula.

7. Bake in the preheated oven for 35-40 minutes or until a toothpick inserted into the center comes out clean.

8. Allow the cake to cool in the pan for 10 minutes, then transfer it to a wire rack to cool completely.

For the Orange Glaze:

1. In a small bowl, whisk together powdered sugar, fresh orange juice, and orange zest until smooth.

2. Once the cake is completely cooled, drizzle the orange glaze over the top.

3. Garnish with chopped pistachios, if desired.

4. Allow the glaze to set before slicing and serving.

Dark Chocolate-Dipped Strawberries

Ingredients:

- 1 pound fresh strawberries, washed and dried
- 8 ounces dark chocolate, chopped
- 1 tablespoon coconut oil or unsalted butter (optional, for smoother dipping)
- Toppings of your choice (chopped nuts, shredded coconut, sprinkles)

Instructions:

1. Line a baking sheet with parchment paper.

2. In a heatproof bowl, combine the chopped dark chocolate and coconut oil or unsalted butter. Melt the chocolate using a double boiler or microwave in short 20-30 second bursts, stirring well between each interval until smooth.

3. Hold each strawberry by the stem and dip it into the melted chocolate, swirling to coat about two-thirds of the berry. Allow any excess chocolate to drip off.

4. If desired, roll the chocolate-covered portion of the strawberry in your choice of toppings, such as chopped nuts, shredded coconut, or sprinkles.

5. Place the dipped strawberries on the prepared baking sheet.

6. Repeat the dipping process for each strawberry.

7. Allow the chocolate-dipped strawberries to cool and set at room temperature or in the refrigerator.

8. If stored in the refrigerator, allow them to come to room temperature for a few minutes before serving.

9. Serve the Dark Chocolate-Dipped Strawberries as a delightful and indulgent treat.

Peach and Oat Crisp

Ingredients:

For the Peach Filling:

- 6-8 ripe peaches, peeled, pitted, and sliced
- 1/2 cup granulated sugar
- 2 tablespoons all-purpose flour
- 1 teaspoon ground cinnamon
- 1 teaspoon vanilla extract
- Zest of 1 lemon

For the Oat Topping:

- 1 cup old-fashioned oats
- 1/2 cup all-purpose flour
- 1/2 cup brown sugar, packed
- 1/2 teaspoon ground cinnamon
- 1/4 teaspoon salt
- 1/2 cup unsalted butter, cold and diced

Instructions:

1. Preheat your oven to 350°F (175°C). Grease a baking dish (9x13 inches or a similar size) with butter or cooking spray.
2. In a large mixing bowl, combine sliced peaches, granulated sugar, all-purpose flour, ground cinnamon, vanilla extract, and lemon zest.

3. Toss the ingredients together until the peaches are well coated.

4. Transfer the peach mixture to the prepared baking dish, spreading it evenly.

5. In a separate bowl, prepare the oat topping. Combine old-fashioned oats, all-purpose flour, brown sugar, ground cinnamon, and salt. Add the cold, diced butter and use a pastry cutter or your fingers to work the butter into the dry ingredients until the mixture resembles coarse crumbs.

6. Sprinkle the oat topping evenly over the peach filling in the baking dish.

7. Bake in the preheated oven for 40-45 minutes or until the peach filling is bubbly, and the oat topping is golden brown.

8. Allow the Peach and Oat Crisp to cool slightly before serving.

9. Serve the crisp warm, optionally topped with a scoop of vanilla ice cream or a dollop of whipped cream.

Vanilla Pomegranate Popsicles

Ingredients:

- 2 cups pomegranate juice
- 1/4 cup honey or maple syrup (adjust to taste)
- 1 teaspoon vanilla extract
- 1/2 cup pomegranate arils (optional, for texture)

Instructions:

1. In a mixing bowl, combine pomegranate juice, honey or maple syrup, and vanilla extract. Stir until the sweetener is fully dissolved.
2. If you prefer popsicles with a bit of texture, add pomegranate arils to the mixture and stir gently.
3. Taste the mixture and adjust the sweetness if necessary.
4. Pour the mixture into popsicle molds, leaving a little space at the top for expansion.
5. Insert popsicle sticks into the molds.
6. Place the molds in the freezer and freeze for about 2-3 hours until the popsicles are partially set.
7. After 2-3 hours, remove the molds from the freezer and insert popsicle sticks into the partially frozen mixture. This helps to keep the sticks in place.

8. Return the molds to the freezer and freeze for an additional 4-6 hours or until the popsicles are completely frozen.

9. Once fully frozen, run the molds under warm water for a few seconds to loosen the popsicles. Gently remove the popsicles from the molds.

10. Serve the Vanilla Pomegranate Popsicles immediately and enjoy this refreshing and naturally sweet treat!

Lemon Blueberry Frozen Yogurt

Ingredients:

- 2 cups fresh or frozen blueberries
- 1/2 cup granulated sugar (adjust to taste)
- 2 tablespoons lemon juice
- 2 cups plain Greek yogurt
- Zest of 1 lemon
- 1 teaspoon vanilla extract

Instructions:

1. In a blender or food processor, combine blueberries, granulated sugar, and lemon juice. Blend until smooth.

2. Strain the blueberry mixture through a fine-mesh sieve to remove seeds and skins, if desired, for a smoother texture. This step is optional based on your preference.

3. In a large mixing bowl, combine Greek yogurt, lemon zest, and vanilla extract.

4. Add the strained blueberry mixture to the yogurt mixture and stir until well combined.

5. Taste the mixture and adjust the sweetness if necessary by adding more sugar.

6. Pour the mixture into an ice cream maker and churn according to the manufacturer's instructions until it reaches a frozen yogurt consistency.

7. Once churned, transfer the Lemon Blueberry Frozen Yogurt to a lidded container.

8. Freeze the frozen yogurt for an additional 2-3 hours to firm up.

9. Before serving, let the frozen yogurt sit at room temperature for a few minutes to soften slightly.

10. Serve the Lemon Blueberry Frozen Yogurt in bowls or cones and enjoy this refreshing and tangy frozen treat!

Almond Flour Banana Bread

Ingredients:

- 3 ripe bananas, mashed
- 3 large eggs
- 1/4 cup coconut oil or melted butter
- 1/4 cup maple syrup or honey
- 1 teaspoon vanilla extract
- 2 1/2 cups almond flour
- 1 teaspoon baking soda
- 1/2 teaspoon salt
- 1 teaspoon ground cinnamon
- 1/2 cup chopped nuts (walnuts or pecans), optional

Instructions:

1. Preheat your oven to 350°F (175°C). Grease a standard-sized loaf pan and line it with parchment paper for easy removal.

2. In a large mixing bowl, mash the ripe bananas with a fork or potato masher.

3. Add the eggs, coconut oil or melted butter, maple syrup or honey, and vanilla extract to the mashed bananas. Mix until well combined.

4. In a separate bowl, whisk together almond flour, baking soda, salt, and ground cinnamon.

5. Gradually add the dry ingredients to the wet ingredients, stirring until just combined.

6. If desired, fold in chopped nuts.

7. Pour the batter into the prepared loaf pan, spreading it evenly.

8. Bake in the preheated oven for 50-60 minutes or until a toothpick inserted into the center comes out clean.

9. Allow the Almond Flour Banana Bread to cool in the pan for 10-15 minutes, then transfer it to a wire rack to cool completely.

10. Once cooled, slice and serve.

Mango Coconut Chia Popsicles

Ingredients:

- 2 ripe mangoes, peeled and diced
- 1 cup coconut milk
- 2 tablespoons chia seeds
- 2-3 tablespoons honey or maple syrup (adjust to taste)
- 1 teaspoon vanilla extract
- Pinch of salt (optional)

Instructions:

1. In a blender, combine diced mangoes, coconut milk, chia seeds, honey or maple syrup, vanilla extract, and a pinch of salt if desired.

2. Blend the mixture until smooth and well combined.

3. Taste the mixture and adjust the sweetness if necessary by adding more honey or maple syrup.

4. Pour the mango coconut chia mixture into popsicle molds, leaving a little space at the top for expansion.

5. Insert popsicle sticks into the molds.

6. Tap the molds gently on the countertop to remove any air bubbles.

7. Place the molds in the freezer and freeze for at least 4-6 hours or until the popsicles are completely frozen.

8. Once fully frozen, run the molds under warm water for a few seconds to loosen the popsicles. Gently remove the popsicles from the molds.

9. Serve the Mango Coconut Chia Popsicles immediately and enjoy this tropical and refreshing frozen treat!

"With each breath, I inhale positivity and exhale negativity."

"My mind and body are in harmony, creating an environment for healing."

CHAPTER 10: SOUP RECIPES

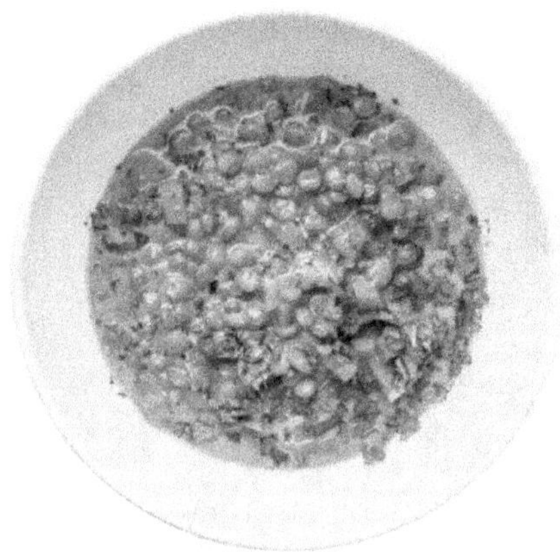

Vegetable and Lentil Soup

Ingredients:

- 1 cup dry green or brown lentils, rinsed and drained
- 2 tablespoons olive oil
- 1 large onion, diced
- 3 cloves garlic, minced
- 2 carrots, peeled and chopped
- 2 celery stalks, chopped
- 1 bell pepper, diced (any color)
- 1 zucchini, diced
- 1 teaspoon ground cumin
- 1 teaspoon ground coriander

- 1 teaspoon smoked paprika
- 1/2 teaspoon turmeric
- 1/4 teaspoon cayenne pepper (optional, for heat)
- 8 cups vegetable broth
- 1 can (14 ounces) diced tomatoes
- 2 bay leaves
- Salt and black pepper to taste
- 3 cups chopped kale or spinach
- Juice of 1 lemon
- Fresh parsley for garnish (optional)

Instructions:

1. In a large pot, heat olive oil over medium heat. Add diced onions and cook until softened, about 5 minutes.

2. Add minced garlic, chopped carrots, celery, bell pepper, and zucchini to the pot. Sauté the vegetables for another 5-7 minutes until they start to soften.

3. Stir in ground cumin, ground coriander, smoked paprika, turmeric, and cayenne pepper (if using). Cook for an additional 1-2 minutes to toast the spices.

4. Add rinsed lentils, vegetable broth, diced tomatoes (with their juice), and bay leaves to the pot.

5. Season with salt and black pepper to taste. Bring the soup to a boil, then reduce the heat to low and let it simmer, covered, for about 25-30 minutes or until the lentils are tender.

6. Stir in chopped kale or spinach and cook for an additional 5 minutes until the greens are wilted.

7. Remove the bay leaves from the soup and discard them.

8. Add lemon juice to the soup and adjust the seasoning if necessary.

9. Serve the Vegetable and Lentil Soup hot, garnished with fresh parsley if desired.

Mushroom and Barley Soup

Ingredients:

- 1 cup pearl barley, rinsed and drained
- 2 tablespoons olive oil
- 1 onion, finely chopped
- 2 carrots, peeled and diced
- 2 celery stalks, diced
- 3 cloves garlic, minced

- 8 ounces mushrooms, sliced (any variety you prefer)
- 1 teaspoon dried thyme
- 1 teaspoon dried rosemary
- 6 cups vegetable or mushroom broth
- 2 bay leaves
- Salt and black pepper to taste
- 1 cup spinach or kale, chopped
- Juice of 1 lemon
- Fresh parsley for garnish (optional)

Instructions:

1. In a medium-sized pot, heat olive oil over medium heat. Add chopped onions, carrots, and celery. Cook until the vegetables are softened, about 5-7 minutes.

2. Add minced garlic and sliced mushrooms to the pot. Cook for an additional 5 minutes until the mushrooms release their moisture.

3. Stir in dried thyme and dried rosemary, and cook for another 2 minutes to allow the herbs to become fragrant.

4. Add rinsed pearl barley to the pot and stir to coat the barley with the vegetables and herbs.

5. Pour in the vegetable or mushroom broth and add bay leaves. Season with salt and black pepper to taste.

6. Bring the soup to a boil, then reduce the heat to low, cover, and let it simmer for about 30-40 minutes or until the barley is tender.

7. Stir in chopped spinach or kale and cook for an additional 5 minutes until the greens are wilted.

8. Remove the bay leaves from the soup and discard them.

9. Add lemon juice to the soup and adjust the seasoning if necessary.

10. Serve the Mushroom and Barley Soup hot, garnished with fresh parsley if desired.

Chicken and Vegetable Quinoa Soup

Ingredients:

- 1 cup quinoa, rinsed and drained
- 1 tablespoon olive oil
- 1 onion, finely chopped
- 3 carrots, peeled and diced
- 3 celery stalks, diced
- 3 cloves garlic, minced

- 1 pound boneless, skinless chicken breasts, diced
- 8 cups chicken broth
- 1 teaspoon dried thyme
- 1 teaspoon dried rosemary
- 1 bay leaf
- Salt and black pepper to taste
- 2 cups broccoli florets
- 1 zucchini, diced
- 1 cup frozen peas
- Juice of 1 lemon
- Fresh parsley for garnish (optional)

Instructions:

1. In a large pot, heat olive oil over medium heat. Add chopped onions, carrots, and celery. Cook until the vegetables are softened, about 5-7 minutes.

2. Add minced garlic and diced chicken to the pot. Cook until the chicken is browned on all sides, about 5 minutes.

3. Pour in chicken broth, add rinsed quinoa, dried thyme, dried rosemary, bay leaf, salt, and black pepper. Stir to combine.

4. Bring the soup to a boil, then reduce the heat to low, cover, and let it simmer for about 15-20 minutes or until the quinoa is cooked and the chicken is fully cooked through.

5. Stir in broccoli florets, diced zucchini, and frozen peas. Cook for an additional 5-7 minutes until the vegetables are tender.

6. Remove the bay leaf from the soup and discard it.

7. Add lemon juice to the soup and adjust the seasoning if necessary.

8. Serve the Chicken and Vegetable Quinoa Soup hot, garnished with fresh parsley if desired.

Spinach and White Bean Soup

Ingredients:

- 2 tablespoons olive oil
- 1 onion, finely chopped
- 3 cloves garlic, minced
- 2 carrots, peeled and diced
- 2 celery stalks, diced
- 1 teaspoon dried thyme
- 1 teaspoon dried rosemary

- 2 cans (15 ounces each) white beans (cannellini or Great Northern), drained and rinsed
- 6 cups vegetable broth or chicken broth
- 1 bay leaf
- Salt and black pepper to taste
- 5 cups fresh spinach, chopped
- Juice of 1 lemon
- Grated Parmesan cheese for serving (optional)

Instructions:

1. In a large pot, heat olive oil over medium heat. Add chopped onions, carrots, and celery. Cook until the vegetables are softened, about 5-7 minutes.

2. Add minced garlic, dried thyme, and dried rosemary to the pot. Cook for an additional 2 minutes until the herbs become fragrant.

3. Stir in white beans, vegetable or chicken broth, and add a bay leaf. Season with salt and black pepper to taste.

4. Bring the soup to a boil, then reduce the heat to low, cover, and let it simmer for about 15-20 minutes to allow the flavors to meld.

5. Add chopped spinach to the soup and cook for an additional 5 minutes until the spinach is wilted.

6. Remove the bay leaf from the soup and discard it.

7. Stir in lemon juice to brighten the flavors. Adjust the seasoning if necessary.

8. Serve the Spinach and White Bean Soup hot, optionally topped with grated Parmesan cheese.

Roasted Butternut Squash Soup

Ingredients:

- 1 large butternut squash, peeled, seeded, and diced (about 4 cups)
- 2 tablespoons olive oil
- 1 onion, chopped
- 2 carrots, peeled and chopped
- 2 celery stalks, chopped
- 3 cloves garlic, minced
- 1 teaspoon ground cumin
- 1/2 teaspoon ground coriander
- 1/2 teaspoon smoked paprika
- 6 cups vegetable broth
- Salt and black pepper to taste

- 1 bay leaf
- 1/2 cup coconut milk or heavy cream
- Fresh parsley or chives for garnish (optional)

Instructions:

1. Preheat your oven to 400°F (200°C).

2. Place the diced butternut squash on a baking sheet. Drizzle with olive oil, season with salt and pepper, and toss to coat evenly. Roast in the preheated oven for about 30-40 minutes or until the squash is tender and caramelized.

3. In a large pot, heat olive oil over medium heat. Add chopped onions, carrots, and celery. Cook until the vegetables are softened, about 5-7 minutes.

4. Add minced garlic, ground cumin, ground coriander, and smoked paprika to the pot. Cook for an additional 2 minutes until the spices become fragrant.

5. Add the roasted butternut squash to the pot, along with vegetable broth and a bay leaf. Bring the soup to a boil, then reduce the heat to low, cover, and let it simmer for about 15-20 minutes.

6. Remove the bay leaf from the soup and discard it.

7. Use an immersion blender to puree the soup until smooth. Alternatively, carefully transfer the soup to a blender in batches and blend until smooth.

8. Stir in coconut milk or heavy cream, and season the soup with salt and black pepper to taste.

9. Heat the soup for an additional 5 minutes, making sure it's heated through.

10. Serve the Roasted Butternut Squash Soup hot, garnished with fresh parsley or chives if desired.

Tomato Basil Chickpea Soup

Ingredients:

- 2 tablespoons olive oil
- 1 onion, chopped
- 3 cloves garlic, minced
- 2 carrots, peeled and diced
- 2 celery stalks, diced
- 1 teaspoon dried oregano
- 1 teaspoon dried basil
- 1/2 teaspoon dried thyme
- 1/4 teaspoon red pepper flakes (optional, for heat)

- 2 cans (15 ounces each) chickpeas, drained and rinsed
- 1 can (28 ounces) crushed tomatoes
- 4 cups vegetable broth
- Salt and black pepper to taste
- 1 bay leaf
- 1/2 cup fresh basil, chopped
- Grated Parmesan cheese for serving (optional)

Instructions:

1. In a large pot, heat olive oil over medium heat. Add chopped onions, carrots, and celery. Cook until the vegetables are softened, about 5-7 minutes.

2. Add minced garlic, dried oregano, dried basil, dried thyme, and red pepper flakes (if using). Cook for an additional 2 minutes until the herbs become fragrant.

3. Stir in chickpeas, crushed tomatoes, vegetable broth, and add a bay leaf. Season with salt and black pepper to taste.

4. Bring the soup to a boil, then reduce the heat to low, cover, and let it simmer for about 20-25 minutes.

5. Remove the bay leaf from the soup and discard it.

6. Stir in fresh basil and cook for an additional 2 minutes until the basil is wilted.

7. Taste the soup and adjust the seasoning if necessary.

8. Serve the Tomato Basil Chickpea Soup hot, optionally topped with grated Parmesan cheese.

Turkey and Vegetable Rice Soup

Ingredients:

- 1 tablespoon olive oil
- 1 onion, finely chopped
- 2 carrots, peeled and diced
- 2 celery stalks, diced
- 3 cloves garlic, minced
- 1 pound ground turkey
- 1 teaspoon dried thyme
- 1 teaspoon dried rosemary
- 1/2 teaspoon dried oregano
- Salt and black pepper to taste
- 1 cup long-grain white rice
- 8 cups chicken broth
- 1 bay leaf

- 2 cups mixed vegetables (peas, corn, green beans)
- Juice of 1 lemon
- Fresh parsley for garnish (optional)

Instructions:

1. In a large pot, heat olive oil over medium heat. Add chopped onions, carrots, and celery. Cook until the vegetables are softened, about 5-7 minutes.

2. Add minced garlic, ground turkey, dried thyme, dried rosemary, dried oregano, salt, and black pepper to the pot. Cook, breaking up the turkey with a spoon, until the turkey is browned and cooked through.

3. Stir in long-grain white rice and cook for an additional 2 minutes to toast the rice slightly.

4. Pour in chicken broth and add a bay leaf. Bring the soup to a boil, then reduce the heat to low, cover, and let it simmer for about 15-20 minutes or until the rice is cooked.

5. Add mixed vegetables to the pot and cook for an additional 5-7 minutes until the vegetables are tender.

6. Remove the bay leaf from the soup and discard it.

7. Stir in lemon juice to brighten the flavors. Adjust the seasoning if necessary.

8. Serve the Turkey and Vegetable Rice Soup hot, garnished with fresh parsley if desired.

Cauliflower and Leek Soup

Ingredients:

- 1 large cauliflower, chopped into florets
- 2 leeks, cleaned and sliced
- 2 tablespoons olive oil
- 3 cloves garlic, minced
- 1 teaspoon dried thyme
- 6 cups vegetable broth
- Salt and black pepper to taste
- 1 bay leaf
- 1 cup potatoes, peeled and diced
- 1/2 cup unsweetened almond milk or regular milk
- Juice of 1 lemon
- Fresh chives for garnish (optional)

Instructions:

1. In a large pot, heat olive oil over medium heat. Add sliced leeks and cook until softened, about 5-7 minutes.

2. Add minced garlic and dried thyme to the pot. Cook for an additional 2 minutes until the garlic becomes fragrant.

3. Stir in cauliflower florets, vegetable broth, salt, black pepper, and add a bay leaf. Bring the soup to a boil, then reduce the heat to low, cover, and let it simmer for about 15-20 minutes or until the cauliflower is tender.

4. Add diced potatoes to the pot and continue to simmer for an additional 10-15 minutes until the potatoes are cooked through.

5. Remove the bay leaf from the soup and discard it.

6. Use an immersion blender to puree the soup until smooth. Alternatively, carefully transfer the soup to a blender in batches and blend until smooth.

7. Stir in almond milk or regular milk to achieve the desired creamy consistency.

8. Add lemon juice to the soup and adjust the seasoning if necessary.

9. Serve the Cauliflower and Leek Soup hot, garnished with fresh chives if desired.

Broccoli and Cheddar Soup (Lightened)

Ingredients:

- 2 tablespoons olive oil
- 1 onion, chopped
- 3 cloves garlic, minced
- 3 cups broccoli florets
- 2 medium carrots, peeled and diced
- 1/4 cup all-purpose flour
- 4 cups low-sodium vegetable broth
- 2 cups unsweetened almond milk or skim milk
- 2 cups shredded sharp cheddar cheese
- Salt and black pepper to taste
- 1/2 teaspoon dried mustard powder
- 1/4 teaspoon cayenne pepper (optional, for heat)
- Chopped green onions or chives for garnish (optional)

Instructions:

1. In a large pot, heat olive oil over medium heat. Add chopped onions and cook until softened, about 5-7 minutes.

2. Add minced garlic, broccoli florets, and diced carrots to the pot. Cook for an additional 5 minutes until the vegetables start to soften.

3. Sprinkle flour over the vegetables and stir well to coat. Cook for 2-3 minutes to remove the raw taste of the flour.

4. Slowly pour in vegetable broth and almond milk while continuously stirring to avoid lumps. Bring the soup to a simmer.

5. Reduce the heat to low and let the soup simmer for about 15-20 minutes or until the vegetables are tender.

6. Use an immersion blender to puree the soup until smooth. Alternatively, carefully transfer the soup to a blender in batches and blend until smooth.

7. Stir in shredded cheddar cheese until melted and smooth.

8. Season the soup with salt, black pepper, dried mustard powder, and cayenne pepper (if using). Adjust the seasoning to your liking.

9. Serve the Broccoli and Cheddar Soup hot, garnished with chopped green onions or chives if desired.

Carrot Ginger Turmeric Soup

Ingredients:

- 2 tablespoons olive oil
- 1 onion, chopped
- 3 cloves garlic, minced
- 1 tablespoon fresh ginger, grated
- 1 teaspoon ground turmeric
- 1 pound carrots, peeled and sliced
- 1 medium potato, peeled and diced
- 4 cups vegetable broth
- Salt and black pepper to taste
- 1 can (14 ounces) coconut milk
- Juice of 1 orange
- Fresh cilantro for garnish (optional)

Instructions:

1. In a large pot, heat olive oil over medium heat. Add chopped onions and cook until softened, about 5-7 minutes.
2. Add minced garlic, grated ginger, and ground turmeric to the pot. Cook for an additional 2 minutes until the spices become fragrant.
3. Stir in sliced carrots and diced potatoes. Cook for 5 minutes, stirring occasionally.
4. Pour in vegetable broth, season with salt and black pepper, and bring the soup to a boil. Reduce the heat to low, cover, and let it simmer for about 15-20 minutes or until the vegetables are tender.
5. Use an immersion blender to puree the soup until smooth. Alternatively, carefully transfer the soup to a blender in batches and blend until smooth.
6. Stir in coconut milk and orange juice. Simmer the soup for an additional 5-7 minutes to heat through.
7. Taste the soup and adjust the seasoning if necessary.

8. Serve the Carrot Ginger Turmeric Soup hot, garnished with fresh cilantro if desired.

Split Pea Soup with Ham

Ingredients:

- 1 pound (about 2 cups) green split peas, rinsed and drained
- 2 tablespoons olive oil
- 1 onion, chopped
- 2 carrots, peeled and diced
- 2 celery stalks, diced
- 3 cloves garlic, minced
- 1 teaspoon dried thyme
- 1 bay leaf
- 8 cups vegetable or chicken broth
- 1 pound ham, diced (ham bone or ham hock can also be used)
- Salt and black pepper to taste
- 1 cup potatoes, peeled and diced
- 2 cups spinach or kale, chopped
- Juice of 1 lemon
- Fresh parsley for garnish (optional)

Instructions:

1. In a large pot, heat olive oil over medium heat. Add chopped onions, carrots, and celery. Cook until the vegetables are softened, about 5-7 minutes.

2. Add minced garlic, dried thyme, and bay leaf to the pot. Cook for an additional 2 minutes until the herbs become fragrant.

3. Stir in green split peas, diced ham, and vegetable or chicken broth. Season with salt and black pepper to taste.

4. Bring the soup to a boil, then reduce the heat to low, cover, and let it simmer for about 45-60 minutes or until the split peas are tender.

5. If using a ham bone or ham hock, remove it from the soup and shred any meat from it. Return the shredded meat to the pot.

6. Add diced potatoes to the pot and continue to simmer for an additional 15-20 minutes or until the potatoes are cooked through.

7. Stir in chopped spinach or kale and cook for an additional 5 minutes until the greens are wilted.

8. Remove the bay leaf from the soup and discard it.

9. Stir in lemon juice to brighten the flavors. Adjust the seasoning if necessary.

10. Serve the Split Pea Soup with Ham hot, garnished with fresh parsley if desired.

Fish and Vegetable Chowder

Ingredients:

- 1 pound white fish filets (such as cod or tilapia), cut into bite-sized pieces
- 2 tablespoons olive oil
- 1 onion, chopped
- 2 carrots, peeled and diced
- 2 celery stalks, diced
- 3 cloves garlic, minced
- 1 teaspoon dried thyme
- 1 bay leaf
- 4 cups fish or vegetable broth
- 2 cups potatoes, peeled and diced
- 1 cup corn kernels (fresh or frozen)
- 1 cup peas (fresh or frozen)
- 2 cups milk
- 1/2 cup heavy cream
- Salt and black pepper to taste
- Fresh parsley for garnish (optional)

Instructions:

1. In a large pot, heat olive oil over medium heat. Add chopped onions, carrots, and celery. Cook until the vegetables are softened, about 5-7 minutes.

2. Add minced garlic, dried thyme, and bay leaf to the pot. Cook for an additional 2 minutes until the herbs become fragrant.

3. Stir in diced potatoes and fish or vegetable broth. Season with salt and black pepper to taste.

4. Bring the soup to a boil, then reduce the heat to low, cover, and let it simmer for about 15-20 minutes or until the potatoes are cooked through.

5. Add corn kernels, peas, milk, and heavy cream to the pot. Simmer for an additional 5-7 minutes to heat through.

6. Gently fold in the bite-sized fish pieces and cook for an additional 5-7 minutes until the fish is opaque and flakes easily.

7. Remove the bay leaf from the soup and discard it. Taste the chowder and adjust the seasoning if necessary.

8. Serve the Fish and Vegetable Chowder hot, garnished with fresh parsley if desired.

CHAPTER 11: FISH RECIPES

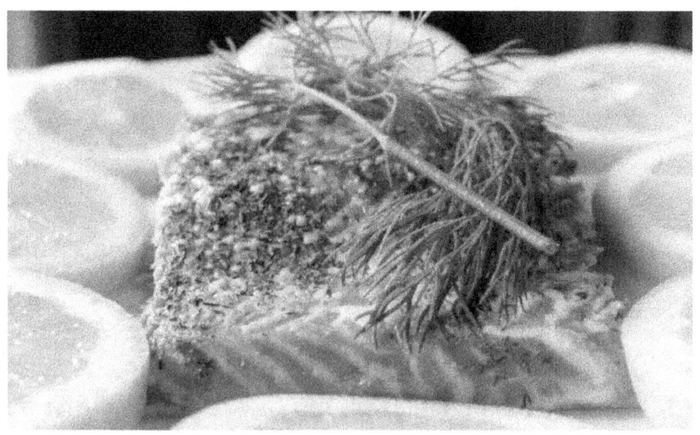

Baked Salmon with Lemon and Dill

Ingredients:

- 4 salmon filets (about 6 ounces each)
- 2 lemons (1 sliced, 1 juiced)
- 2 tablespoons olive oil
- 2 cloves garlic, minced
- 1 tablespoon fresh dill, chopped
- Salt and pepper to taste
- Optional: 1 teaspoon honey for a touch of sweetness

Instructions:

1. Preheat your oven to 375°F (190°C).

2. Place the salmon filets on a baking sheet lined with parchment paper or lightly greased.

3. In a small bowl, mix together the olive oil, minced garlic, fresh dill, lemon juice, salt, and pepper. If you prefer a touch of sweetness, add honey to the mixture and stir well.

4. Brush the salmon filets with the prepared lemon-dill mixture, ensuring each filet is evenly coated.

5. Lay lemon slices on top of each salmon filet for added flavor.

6. Bake in the preheated oven for about 15-20 minutes, or until the salmon flakes easily with a fork. Cooking time may vary based on the thickness of the filets.

7. Once baked, remove from the oven and let it rest for a few minutes before serving.

8. Garnish with additional fresh dill and lemon slices if desired.

Grilled Tilapia with Herb Marinade

Ingredients:

- 4 tilapia filets

- 2 tablespoons olive oil

- 2 tablespoons fresh lemon juice

- 2 cloves garlic, minced

- 1 tablespoon fresh parsley, chopped

- 1 tablespoon fresh cilantro, chopped

- 1 teaspoon dried oregano

- Salt and pepper to taste

- Lemon wedges for serving

Instructions:

1. In a bowl, whisk together the olive oil, lemon juice, minced garlic, chopped parsley, chopped cilantro, dried oregano, salt, and pepper to create the herb marinade.

2. Place the tilapia filets in a shallow dish or a zip-top bag.

3. Pour the herb marinade over the tilapia, ensuring each filet is well-coated. Marinate in the refrigerator for at least 30 minutes, allowing the flavors to infuse.

4. Preheat your grill to medium-high heat.

5. Remove the tilapia from the marinade and let any excess drip off.

6. Grill the tilapia filets for about 3-4 minutes per side, or until the fish is opaque and easily flakes with a fork.

7. While grilling, you can baste the filets with any leftover marinade for added flavor.

8. Once done, remove from the grill and serve hot with lemon wedges on the side.

Cod with Tomato Basil Salsa

Ingredients:

- 4 cod filets
- 2 tablespoons olive oil
- Salt and pepper to taste

Tomato Basil Salsa:

- 2 cups cherry tomatoes, halved
- 1/4 cup fresh basil, thinly sliced
- 1 clove garlic, minced
- 2 tablespoons red onion, finely chopped
- 1 tablespoon balsamic vinegar
- 2 tablespoons extra-virgin olive oil
- Salt and pepper to taste

Instructions:

1. Preheat your oven to 400°F (200°C).

2. Place the cod filets on a baking sheet lined with parchment paper or lightly greased. Drizzle with olive oil and season with salt and pepper.

3. Bake the cod filets in the preheated oven for 12-15 minutes or until the fish is cooked through and flakes easily.

4. While the cod is baking, prepare the tomato basil salsa. In a bowl, combine cherry tomatoes, fresh basil, minced garlic, chopped red onion, balsamic vinegar, extra-virgin olive oil, salt, and pepper. Mix well to combine.

5. Once the cod is done, spoon the tomato basil salsa over the filets.

6. Serve the cod with additional salsa on the side and garnish with extra fresh basil if desired.

Poached Halibut with Ginger and Garlic

Ingredients:

- 4 halibut filets
- 2 cups fish or vegetable broth
- 1/4 cup soy sauce
- 2 tablespoons rice vinegar

- 1 tablespoon fresh ginger, grated

- 2 cloves garlic, minced

- 2 green onions, thinly sliced

- 1 tablespoon sesame oil

- Salt and pepper to taste

- Optional: Red pepper flakes for a hint of spice

Instructions:

1. In a wide skillet or shallow pan, combine fish or vegetable broth, soy sauce, rice vinegar, grated ginger, minced garlic, sliced green onions, sesame oil, salt, and pepper. If you like it spicy, add red pepper flakes to taste.

2. Bring the broth mixture to a gentle simmer over medium heat.

3. Carefully place the halibut filets into the simmering broth.

4. Poach the halibut for about 8-10 minutes, or until the fish is opaque and flakes easily with a fork.

5. While poaching, spoon some of the broth over the filets occasionally for added flavor.

6. Once the halibut is cooked, carefully transfer the filets to serving plates.

7. Drizzle some of the poaching broth over the halibut and garnish with additional sliced green onions.

8. Serve hot, and you can pair it with steamed rice or your choice of side.

Lemon Herb Mahi-Mahi

Ingredients:

- 4 mahi-mahi filets
- 2 tablespoons olive oil
- Zest of 1 lemon
- Juice of 2 lemons
- 2 cloves garlic, minced
- 1 tablespoon fresh thyme, chopped
- 1 tablespoon fresh parsley, chopped
- Salt and pepper to taste

Instructions:

1. Preheat your oven to 400°F (200°C).

2. In a small bowl, mix together olive oil, lemon zest, lemon juice, minced garlic, chopped thyme, chopped parsley, salt, and pepper to create the herb marinade.

3. Place the mahi-mahi filets in a baking dish.

4. Pour the herb marinade over the mahi-mahi, making sure each filet is evenly coated. Allow it to marinate for at least 15-20 minutes.

5. Bake the mahi-mahi in the preheated oven for about 15-20 minutes or until the fish is opaque and flakes easily.

6. Optionally, you can broil the filets for an additional 2-3 minutes for a golden finish.

7. Once done, remove from the oven and serve hot, garnished with additional fresh herbs and lemon slices.

Trout Almondine

Ingredients:

- 4 trout filets
- Salt and pepper to taste
- 1/2 cup all-purpose flour, for dredging
- 4 tablespoons unsalted butter
- 1/4 cup sliced almonds
- 2 tablespoons fresh lemon juice
- 1 tablespoon capers, drained
- 2 tablespoons fresh parsley, chopped
- Lemon wedges for serving

Instructions:

1. Season the trout filets with salt and pepper.

2. Dredge each filet in flour, shaking off any excess.

3. In a large skillet over medium heat, melt 2 tablespoons of butter.

4. Add the trout filets to the skillet and cook for about 3-4 minutes per side or until golden brown and cooked through. Transfer the cooked filets to a serving platter.

5. In the same skillet, add the remaining 2 tablespoons of butter. Allow it to melt and begin to brown slightly.

6. Add the sliced almonds to the browned butter and cook for 1-2 minutes until the almonds are toasted, stirring constantly.

7. Stir in the fresh lemon juice and capers into the almond-butter mixture. Cook for an additional minute, allowing the flavors to combine.

8. Pour the almondine sauce over the trout filets.

9. Garnish with chopped fresh parsley and serve hot, accompanied by lemon wedges.

Miso-Glazed Chilean Sea Bass

Ingredients:

- 4 Chilean sea bass filets
- 1/4 cup white miso paste
- 2 tablespoons mirin (Japanese sweet rice wine)
- 2 tablespoons sake
- 2 tablespoons soy sauce
- 2 tablespoons brown sugar
- 1 tablespoon sesame oil
- 1 tablespoon fresh ginger, grated
- 2 cloves garlic, minced
- Sesame seeds and chopped green onions for garnish

Instructions:

1. Preheat your oven to 400°F (200°C).

2. In a bowl, whisk together white miso paste, mirin, sake, soy sauce, brown sugar, sesame oil, grated ginger, and minced garlic to create the miso glaze.

3. Place the Chilean sea bass filets in a shallow dish and generously coat them with the miso glaze. Allow them to marinate for at least 30 minutes, allowing the flavors to meld.

4. Heat an oven-safe skillet or cast-iron pan over medium-high heat.

5. Place the sea bass filets in the hot skillet, searing each side for about 2 minutes or until browned.

6. Transfer the skillet to the preheated oven and bake for approximately 10-12 minutes or until the sea bass is cooked through and flakes easily with a fork.

7. While baking, baste the filets with the miso glaze from the skillet a couple of times for extra flavor.

8. Once done, garnish the Miso-Glazed Chilean Sea Bass with sesame seeds and chopped green onions.

Steamed Snapper with Vegetables

Ingredients:

- 4 red snapper filets
- Salt and pepper to taste
- 1 tablespoon soy sauce
- 1 tablespoon sesame oil
- 2 tablespoons rice vinegar
- 1 tablespoon fresh ginger, julienned

- 2 cloves garlic, minced
- 1 cup broccoli florets
- 1 medium carrot, julienned
- 1 red bell pepper, thinly sliced
- 1 tablespoon vegetable oil
- Sesame seeds and chopped green onions for garnish

Instructions:

1. Season the snapper filets with salt and pepper.
2. In a small bowl, mix soy sauce, sesame oil, rice vinegar, julienned ginger, and minced garlic to create a marinade.
3. Place each snapper filet on a separate piece of parchment paper or foil. Pour a portion of the marinade over each filet.
4. Arrange the broccoli florets, julienned carrot, and sliced red bell pepper around the snapper filets.
5. Drizzle vegetable oil over the vegetables and season with salt and pepper.
6. Fold the parchment paper or foil to create sealed packets.

7. Steam the packets in a steamer or bamboo steamer for about 12-15 minutes, or until the snapper is opaque and flakes easily.

8. Carefully open the packets, transfer the snapper and vegetables to serving plates.

9. Drizzle any remaining juices from the packets over the fish and vegetables.

10. Garnish with sesame seeds and chopped green onions.

Herb-Crusted Haddock

Ingredients:

- 4 haddock filets
- 1/2 cup breadcrumbs (preferably panko)
- 2 tablespoons fresh parsley, finely chopped
- 1 tablespoon fresh dill, finely chopped
- 1 tablespoon fresh chives, finely chopped
- Zest of 1 lemon
- 2 tablespoons grated Parmesan cheese
- 2 tablespoons Dijon mustard
- 2 tablespoons mayonnaise
- Salt and pepper to taste
- Lemon wedges for serving

Instructions:

1. Preheat your oven to 400°F (200°C).

2. In a bowl, combine breadcrumbs, chopped parsley, chopped dill, chopped chives, lemon zest, and grated Parmesan cheese to create the herb crust.

3. In a separate bowl, mix Dijon mustard and mayonnaise.

4. Season the haddock filets with salt and pepper.

5. Spread a thin layer of the Dijon-mayo mixture over each haddock filet.

6. Press the herb crust onto the coated side of each filet, ensuring an even coating.

7. Place the haddock filets on a baking sheet lined with parchment paper.

8. Bake in the preheated oven for about 12-15 minutes or until the fish is cooked through and the crust is golden brown.

9. Once done, serve hot with lemon wedges on the side.

CHAPTER 12: SMOOTHIES

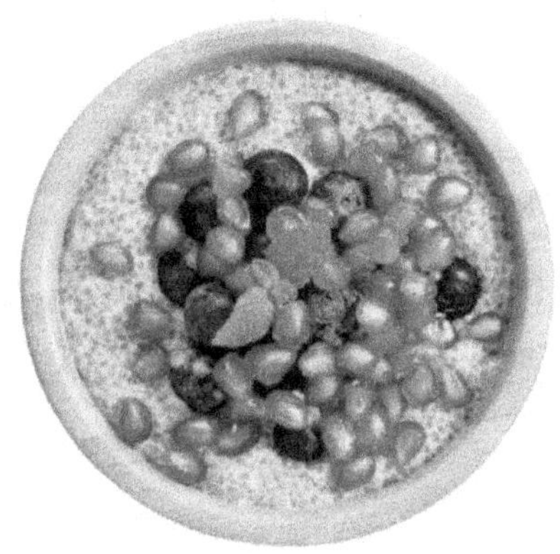

Green Goddess Smoothie

Ingredients:

- 1 cup fresh spinach leaves
- 1/2 cucumber, peeled and sliced
- 1/2 avocado, peeled and pitted
- 1/2 banana
- 1/2 cup plain Greek yogurt
- 1/2 cup coconut water or almond milk
- 1 tablespoon chia seeds
- 1 tablespoon honey or maple syrup (optional for sweetness)
- Ice cubes (optional)

Instructions:

1. Place fresh spinach, sliced cucumber, avocado, banana, Greek yogurt, chia seeds, and coconut water (or almond milk) in a blender.

2. If you desire additional sweetness, add honey or maple syrup to taste.

3. Blend all the ingredients until smooth and creamy. If the smoothie is too thick, you can add more coconut water or almond milk until you achieve your desired consistency.

4. If you prefer a colder smoothie, add a handful of ice cubes and blend again until well combined.

5. Pour the Green Goddess Smoothie into a glass and enjoy immediately.

Berry Blast Smoothie

Ingredients:

- 1 cup mixed berries (strawberries, blueberries, raspberries)
- 1/2 banana
- 1/2 cup Greek yogurt (plain or vanilla)
- 1/2 cup almond milk or any milk of your choice
- 1 tablespoon chia seeds

- 1 tablespoon honey or maple syrup (optional for sweetness)
- Ice cubes (optional)

Instructions:

1. Place mixed berries, banana, Greek yogurt, almond milk (or your preferred milk), chia seeds, and honey (if using) in a blender.
2. If you want a colder smoothie, add a handful of ice cubes.
3. Blend all the ingredients until smooth and well combined. If the smoothie is too thick, you can adjust the consistency by adding more milk.
4. Taste the smoothie and adjust the sweetness by adding more honey or maple syrup if desired.
5. Once everything is blended to your liking, pour the Berry Blast Smoothie into a glass.
6. Garnish with extra berries on top if you'd like.
7. Enjoy this vibrant and delicious smoothie filled with the goodness of mixed berries!

Tropical Turmeric Smoothie

Ingredients:

- 1 cup frozen pineapple chunks
- 1/2 frozen banana

- 1/2 cup mango chunks (fresh or frozen)
- 1/2 cup plain Greek yogurt
- 1/2 teaspoon ground turmeric
- 1/2 teaspoon grated ginger
- 1 tablespoon chia seeds
- 1 tablespoon honey or maple syrup (optional for sweetness)
- 1 cup coconut water or coconut milk
- Ice cubes (optional)

Instructions:

1. In a blender, combine frozen pineapple chunks, frozen banana, mango chunks, Greek yogurt, ground turmeric, grated ginger, chia seeds, and honey (if using).
2. Pour in coconut water or coconut milk to the blender.
3. If you prefer a colder smoothie, add ice cubes.
4. Blend all the ingredients until smooth and creamy. Adjust the consistency by adding more coconut water or coconut milk if needed.
5. Taste the smoothie and adjust the sweetness by adding more honey or maple syrup if desired.
6. Once blended to your liking, pour the Tropical Turmeric Smoothie into a glass.

7. Optionally, garnish with a sprinkle of chia seeds or a slice of pineapple.

8. Enjoy this refreshing and tropical-inspired smoothie with the added benefits of turmeric and ginger!

Citrus Sunshine Smoothie

Ingredients:

- 1 orange, peeled and segmented
- 1/2 grapefruit, peeled and segmented
- 1/2 banana
- 1/2 cup plain Greek yogurt
- 1 tablespoon chia seeds
- 1 tablespoon honey or maple syrup (optional for sweetness)
- 1/2 cup orange juice
- Ice cubes (optional)

Instructions:

1. In a blender, combine orange segments, grapefruit segments, banana, Greek yogurt, chia seeds, and honey (if using).

2. Pour in orange juice to the blender.

3. If you prefer a colder smoothie, add ice cubes.

4. Blend all the ingredients until smooth and well combined. Adjust the consistency by adding more orange juice if needed.

5. Taste the smoothie and adjust the sweetness by adding more honey or maple syrup if desired.

6. Once blended to your liking, pour the Citrus Sunshine Smoothie into a glass.

7. Optionally, garnish with a slice of orange or grapefruit on the rim of the glass.

8. Enjoy this refreshing and vitamin C-packed smoothie that brings the bright flavors of citrus to your day!

Antioxidant Powerhouse Smoothie

Ingredients:

- 1 cup mixed berries (blueberries, strawberries, raspberries)
- 1/2 cup pomegranate seeds
- 1/2 cup spinach leaves
- 1/2 avocado, peeled and pitted
- 1/2 banana
- 1/2 cup Greek yogurt (plain or vanilla)
- 1 tablespoon chia seeds

- 1 tablespoon honey or maple syrup (optional for sweetness)
- 1 cup almond milk or any milk of your choice
- Ice cubes (optional)

Instructions:

1. In a blender, combine mixed berries, pomegranate seeds, spinach leaves, avocado, banana, Greek yogurt, chia seeds, and honey (if using).
2. Pour in almond milk (or your preferred milk) to the blender.
3. If you want a colder smoothie, add a handful of ice cubes.
4. Blend all the ingredients until smooth and well combined. Adjust the consistency by adding more milk if needed.
5. Taste the smoothie and adjust the sweetness by adding more honey or maple syrup if desired.
6. Once blended to your liking, pour the Antioxidant Powerhouse Smoothie into a glass.
7. Optionally, garnish with a sprinkle of chia seeds or a few pomegranate seeds on top.

8. Enjoy this vibrant and nutrient-packed smoothie that's loaded with antioxidants and essential vitamins!

Creamy Avocado Lime Smoothie

Ingredients:

- 1 ripe avocado, peeled and pitted
- 1 banana
- 1 cup spinach leaves
- Juice of 2 limes
- 1/2 cup Greek yogurt (plain or vanilla)
- 1 tablespoon chia seeds
- 1-2 tablespoons honey or maple syrup (adjust to taste)
- 1 cup almond milk or any milk of your choice
- Ice cubes (optional)

Instructions:

1. In a blender, combine the ripe avocado, banana, spinach leaves, lime juice, Greek yogurt, chia seeds, and honey (or maple syrup).
2. Pour in almond milk (or your preferred milk) to the blender.
3. If you want a colder smoothie, add a handful of ice cubes.

4. Blend all the ingredients until smooth and creamy. Adjust the consistency by adding more milk if needed.

5. Taste the smoothie and adjust the sweetness by adding more honey or maple syrup if desired.

6. Once blended to your liking, pour the Creamy Avocado Lime Smoothie into a glass.

7. Optionally, garnish with a slice of lime on the rim of the glass or a sprinkle of chia seeds on top.

8. Enjoy this luscious and refreshing smoothie that combines the creamy richness of avocado with the zesty kick of lime!

Protein-Packed Peanut Butter Banana Smoothie

Ingredients:

- 1 banana
- 2 tablespoons peanut butter
- 1/2 cup Greek yogurt (plain or vanilla)
- 1 scoop protein powder (vanilla or chocolate)
- 1 tablespoon chia seeds
- 1-2 tablespoons honey or maple syrup (adjust to taste)

- 1 cup almond milk or any milk of your choice
- Ice cubes (optional)

Instructions:

1. In a blender, combine the banana, peanut butter, Greek yogurt, protein powder, chia seeds, and honey (or maple syrup).
2. Pour in almond milk (or your preferred milk) to the blender.
3. If you want a colder smoothie, add a handful of ice cubes.
4. Blend all the ingredients until smooth and well combined. Adjust the consistency by adding more milk if needed.
5. Taste the smoothie and adjust the sweetness by adding more honey or maple syrup if desired.
6. Once blended to your liking, pour the Protein-Packed Peanut Butter Banana Smoothie into a glass.
7. Optionally, drizzle a bit of peanut butter on top for extra flavor.
8. Enjoy this delicious and protein-rich smoothie that combines the classic combination of peanut butter and banana for a satisfying and energizing drink!

Beetroot and Berry Bliss Smoothie

Ingredients:

- 1 small beetroot, peeled and diced
- 1 cup mixed berries (strawberries, blueberries, raspberries)
- 1/2 banana
- 1/2 cup Greek yogurt (plain or vanilla)
- 1 tablespoon chia seeds
- 1-2 tablespoons honey or maple syrup (adjust to taste)
- 1 cup coconut water or any liquid of your choice
- Ice cubes (optional)

Instructions:

1. In a blender, combine diced beetroot, mixed berries, banana, Greek yogurt, chia seeds, and honey (or maple syrup).
2. Pour in coconut water (or your preferred liquid) to the blender.
3. If you want a colder smoothie, add a handful of ice cubes.
4. Blend all the ingredients until smooth and well combined. Adjust the consistency by adding more liquid if needed.

5. Taste the smoothie and adjust the sweetness by adding more honey or maple syrup if desired.

6. Once blended to your liking, pour the Beetroot and Berry Bliss Smoothie into a glass.

7. Optionally, garnish with a few whole berries or a sprinkle of chia seeds on top.

8. Enjoy this vibrant and nutrient-packed smoothie that combines the earthy flavors of beetroot with the sweetness of mixed berries!

Minty Pineapple Kale Smoothie

Ingredients:

- 1 cup fresh pineapple chunks
- 1 cup kale leaves, stems removed
- 1/2 banana
- 1/4 cup fresh mint leaves
- 1/2 cup Greek yogurt (plain or vanilla)
- 1 tablespoon chia seeds
- 1-2 tablespoons honey or maple syrup (adjust to taste)
- 1 cup coconut water or any liquid of your choice
- Ice cubes (optional)

Instructions:

1. In a blender, combine fresh pineapple chunks, kale leaves, banana, fresh mint leaves, Greek yogurt, chia seeds, and honey (or maple syrup).
2. Pour in coconut water (or your preferred liquid) to the blender.
3. If you want a colder smoothie, add a handful of ice cubes.
4. Blend all the ingredients until smooth and well combined. Adjust the consistency by adding more liquid if needed.
5. Taste the smoothie and adjust the sweetness by adding more honey or maple syrup if desired.
6. Once blended to your liking, pour the Minty Pineapple Kale Smoothie into a glass.
7. Optionally, garnish with a sprig of fresh mint on the rim of the glass.
8. Enjoy this refreshing and minty green smoothie that combines the sweetness of pineapple with the vibrant flavors of kale and mint!

Cherry Almond Delight Smoothie

Ingredients:

- 1 cup frozen cherries, pitted

- 1/2 banana
- 1/4 cup almonds, preferably soaked
- 1/2 cup Greek yogurt (plain or vanilla)
- 1 tablespoon chia seeds
- 1-2 tablespoons honey or maple syrup (adjust to taste)
- 1 cup almond milk or any liquid of your choice
- Ice cubes (optional)

Instructions:

1. In a blender, combine frozen cherries, banana, soaked almonds, Greek yogurt, chia seeds, and honey (or maple syrup).
2. Pour in almond milk (or your preferred liquid) to the blender.
3. If you want a colder smoothie, add a handful of ice cubes.
4. Blend all the ingredients until smooth and well combined. Adjust the consistency by adding more liquid if needed.
5. Taste the smoothie and adjust the sweetness by adding more honey or maple syrup if desired.
6. Once blended to your liking, pour the Cherry Almond Delight Smoothie into a glass.

7. Optionally, garnish with a few whole cherries or a sprinkle of sliced almonds on top.

8. Enjoy this rich and nutty smoothie that combines the sweet-tart flavor of cherries with the crunch of almonds!

Detoxifying Green Tea Smoothie

Ingredients:

- 1 cup brewed green tea, cooled
- 1/2 cucumber, peeled and sliced
- 1/2 lemon, peeled and segmented
- 1 cup kale leaves, stems removed
- 1/2 banana
- 1 tablespoon chia seeds
- 1-2 tablespoons honey or maple syrup (adjust to taste)
- Ice cubes (optional)

Instructions:

1. Brew green tea and allow it to cool to room temperature.

2. In a blender, combine cooled green tea, sliced cucumber, segmented lemon, kale leaves, banana, chia seeds, and honey (or maple syrup).

3. If you want a colder smoothie, add a handful of ice cubes.

4. Blend all the ingredients until smooth and well combined. Adjust the consistency by adding more liquid if needed.

5. Taste the smoothie and adjust the sweetness by adding more honey or maple syrup if desired.

6. Once blended to your liking, pour the Detoxifying Green Tea Smoothie into a glass.

7. Optionally, garnish with a slice of cucumber or a lemon wedge on the rim of the glass.

8. Enjoy this refreshing and detoxifying smoothie that combines the antioxidant power of green tea with the cleansing properties of cucumber and lemon!

Blueberry Lavender Relaxation Smoothie

Ingredients:

- 1 cup blueberries (fresh or frozen)
- 1/2 banana
- 1/2 cup plain Greek yogurt
- 1 tablespoon dried culinary lavender buds
- 1 tablespoon chia seeds

- 1-2 tablespoons honey or maple syrup (adjust to taste)
- 1 cup almond milk or any milk of your choice
- Ice cubes (optional)

Instructions:

1. In a blender, combine blueberries, banana, Greek yogurt, dried lavender buds, chia seeds, and honey (or maple syrup).
2. Pour in almond milk (or your preferred milk) to the blender.
3. If you want a colder smoothie, add a handful of ice cubes.
4. Blend all the ingredients until smooth and well combined. Adjust the consistency by adding more liquid if needed.
5. Taste the smoothie and adjust the sweetness by adding more honey or maple syrup if desired.
6. Once blended to your liking, pour the Blueberry Lavender Relaxation Smoothie into a glass.
7. Optionally, garnish with a sprinkle of dried lavender buds on top.
8. Enjoy this calming and aromatic smoothie that combines the sweet flavor of blueberries with the soothing essence of lavender!

Peach Ginger Turmeric Smoothie

Ingredients:

- 1 cup frozen or fresh peach slices
- 1/2 banana
- 1 teaspoon fresh ginger, grated
- 1/2 teaspoon ground turmeric
- 1/2 cup Greek yogurt (plain or vanilla)
- 1 tablespoon chia seeds
- 1-2 tablespoons honey or maple syrup (adjust to taste)
- 1 cup coconut water or any liquid of your choice
- Ice cubes (optional)

Instructions:

1. In a blender, combine peach slices, banana, grated ginger, ground turmeric, Greek yogurt, chia seeds, and honey (or maple syrup).
2. Pour in coconut water (or your preferred liquid) to the blender.
3. If you want a colder smoothie, add a handful of ice cubes.
4. Blend all the ingredients until smooth and well combined. Adjust the consistency by adding more liquid if needed.

5. Taste the smoothie and adjust the sweetness by adding more honey or maple syrup if desired.

6. Once blended to your liking, pour the Peach Ginger Turmeric Smoothie into a glass.

7. Optionally, garnish with a slice of peach or a sprinkle of ground turmeric on top.

8. Enjoy this vibrant and immune-boosting smoothie that combines the sweetness of peaches with the warmth of ginger and turmeric!

Mango Coconut Energizer Smoothie

Ingredients:

- 1 cup fresh or frozen mango chunks
- 1/2 banana
- 1/4 cup shredded coconut
- 1/2 cup Greek yogurt (plain or vanilla)
- 1 tablespoon chia seeds
- 1-2 tablespoons honey or maple syrup (adjust to taste)
- 1 cup coconut water or any liquid of your choice
- Ice cubes (optional)

Instructions:

1. In a blender, combine mango chunks, banana, shredded coconut, Greek yogurt, chia seeds, and honey (or maple syrup).

2. Pour in coconut water (or your preferred liquid) to the blender.

3. If you want a colder smoothie, add a handful of ice cubes.

4. Blend all the ingredients until smooth and well combined. Adjust the consistency by adding more liquid if needed.

5. Taste the smoothie and adjust the sweetness by adding more honey or maple syrup if desired.

6. Once blended to your liking, pour the Mango Coconut Energizer Smoothie into a glass.

7. Optionally, garnish with a sprinkle of shredded coconut on top.

8. Enjoy this tropical and refreshing smoothie that combines the luscious taste of mango with the tropical twist of coconut!

CHAPTER 13: HERBS AND SPICES

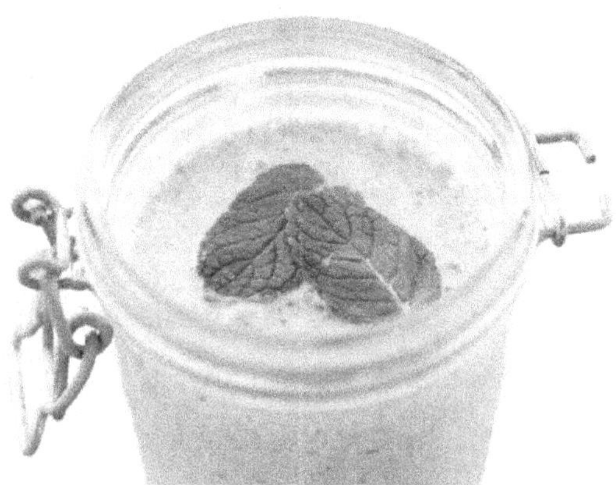

Turmeric-Roasted Vegetables

Ingredients:

- Assorted vegetables (e.g., carrots, cauliflower, broccoli, sweet potatoes, Brussels sprouts), washed and chopped
- 2 tablespoons olive oil
- 1 teaspoon ground turmeric
- 1 teaspoon cumin
- 1 teaspoon paprika
- Salt and pepper to taste
- Optional: garlic powder or minced garlic for added flavor

Instructions:

1. Preheat your oven to 400°F (200°C).

2. In a large mixing bowl, combine the chopped vegetables with olive oil, turmeric, cumin, paprika, salt, and pepper. Toss the vegetables until they are evenly coated with the spices and oil.

3. If you're using minced garlic, add it to the vegetable mixture and mix well.

4. Spread the seasoned vegetables in a single layer on a baking sheet. Make sure not to overcrowd the pan to allow even roasting.

5. Roast the vegetables in the preheated oven for 25-30 minutes or until they are tender and golden brown. You may want to toss the vegetables halfway through the cooking time for even roasting.

6. Once the vegetables are done, remove them from the oven and let them cool slightly before serving.

7. Garnish with fresh herbs like parsley or cilantro if desired.

Ginger-Infused Quinoa

Ingredients:

- 1 cup quinoa, rinsed thoroughly
- 2 cups water or vegetable broth
- 1 tablespoon olive oil
- 1 tablespoon fresh ginger, finely grated
- 1 clove garlic, minced
- Salt and pepper to taste
- Optional: chopped green onions or cilantro for garnish

Instructions:

1. Rinse the quinoa under cold water to remove any bitterness.

2. In a medium saucepan, heat olive oil over medium heat. Add the grated ginger and minced garlic, sautéing for 1-2 minutes until fragrant.

3. Add the rinsed quinoa to the saucepan and stir to coat the grains with the ginger and garlic-infused oil.

4. Pour in the water or vegetable broth and add salt and pepper to taste. Bring the mixture to a boil.

5. Once boiling, reduce the heat to low, cover the saucepan with a lid, and simmer for about 15 minutes or until the quinoa has absorbed the liquid and is tender.

6. Remove the saucepan from heat and let it sit, covered, for an additional 5 minutes to allow the quinoa to steam.

7. Fluff the quinoa with a fork and transfer it to a serving dish.

8. Garnish with chopped green onions or cilantro if desired.

Basil Pesto with Walnuts

Ingredients:

- 2 cups fresh basil leaves, washed and packed
- 1/2 cup walnuts, toasted
- 1/2 cup grated Parmesan cheese
- 3 cloves garlic, peeled
- 1/2 teaspoon salt
- 1/4 teaspoon black pepper
- 1 cup extra-virgin olive oil

Instructions:

1. Toast the walnuts in a dry pan over medium heat until they become fragrant. Be careful not to burn them. Set aside to cool.

2. In a food processor, combine the fresh basil, toasted walnuts, grated Parmesan cheese, garlic, salt, and black pepper.

3. Pulse the ingredients a few times to break them down.

4. With the food processor running, slowly drizzle in the olive oil through the feed tube. Continue processing until the mixture reaches your desired consistency. You may need to stop and scrape down the sides of the processor bowl to ensure even blending.

5. Taste the pesto and adjust the salt and pepper if necessary. If you prefer a thinner consistency, you can add more olive oil and blend again.

6. Once the pesto reaches your desired taste and texture, transfer it to a jar or airtight container.

7. Store the basil pesto in the refrigerator. It can be used immediately or kept for a few days. For longer storage, consider freezing it in ice cube trays for easy portioning.

Cumin-Spiced Lentil Soup

Ingredients:

- 1 cup dried lentils, rinsed and drained
- 1 large onion, finely chopped
- 3 cloves garlic, minced
- 2 carrots, diced
- 2 celery stalks, diced
- 1 can (14 oz) diced tomatoes
- 6 cups vegetable or chicken broth
- 1 teaspoon ground cumin
- 1 teaspoon ground coriander
- 1/2 teaspoon smoked paprika
- 1/2 teaspoon turmeric
- Salt and pepper to taste
- 2 tablespoons olive oil
- Fresh cilantro or parsley for garnish (optional)
- Lemon wedges for serving

Instructions:

1. In a large pot, heat olive oil over medium heat. Add chopped onions and sauté until they become translucent.
2. Add minced garlic and sauté for an additional minute until fragrant.

3. Stir in ground cumin, ground coriander, smoked paprika, and turmeric. Cook for another minute to toast the spices.

4. Add diced carrots and celery to the pot. Cook for 5 minutes, stirring occasionally.

5. Pour in the rinsed lentils, diced tomatoes (with their juices), and broth. Season with salt and pepper to taste.

6. Bring the soup to a boil, then reduce the heat to low, cover, and simmer for about 25-30 minutes or until the lentils are tender.

7. Adjust the seasoning if needed and add more broth if you prefer a thinner soup.

8. Serve the cumin-spiced lentil soup hot, garnished with fresh cilantro or parsley if desired. Offer lemon wedges on the side for a burst of citrus flavor.

Rosemary and Lemon Grilled Chicken

Ingredients:

- 4 boneless, skinless chicken breasts
- 2 tablespoons olive oil
- Zest and juice of 1 lemon
- 2 tablespoons fresh rosemary, finely chopped

- 3 cloves garlic, minced

- 1 teaspoon Dijon mustard

- Salt and pepper to taste

Instructions:

1. In a small bowl, whisk together olive oil, lemon zest, lemon juice, chopped rosemary, minced garlic, Dijon mustard, salt, and pepper. This mixture will be your marinade.

2. Place the chicken breasts in a resealable plastic bag or shallow dish.

3. Pour half of the marinade over the chicken, making sure each piece is coated. Reserve the remaining marinade for later.

4. Seal the bag or cover the dish and refrigerate the chicken for at least 30 minutes to marinate. For a richer flavor, you can marinate it for up to 24 hours.

5. Preheat the grill to medium-high heat.

6. Remove the chicken from the refrigerator and let it come to room temperature for about 10 minutes.

7. Grease the grill grates to prevent sticking.

8. Grill the chicken breasts for 6-8 minutes per side, or until they reach an internal temperature of 165°F (74°C) and have nice grill marks.

9. During the last few minutes of grilling, baste the chicken with the reserved marinade for added flavor.

10. Once cooked through, transfer the grilled chicken to a serving platter and let it rest for a few minutes.

11. Garnish with additional fresh rosemary and lemon slices if desired.

Minty Green Smoothie

Ingredients:

- 1 cup fresh spinach leaves, washed
- 1/2 cup fresh mint leaves, washed
- 1/2 cucumber, peeled and sliced
- 1 green apple, cored and chopped
- 1/2 avocado, peeled and pitted
- 1 cup coconut water or water
- 1 tablespoon chia seeds (optional)
- Ice cubes (optional)
- Honey or agave syrup to sweeten (optional)

Instructions:

1. In a blender, combine fresh spinach, mint leaves, cucumber slices, chopped green apple, and avocado.

2. Add coconut water or water to the blender to help with blending. If you prefer a colder smoothie, you can also add ice cubes.

3. Optionally, add chia seeds for an extra boost of nutrition. Chia seeds will add thickness to the smoothie and provide omega-3 fatty acids.

4. Blend all the ingredients until smooth and creamy. If the consistency is too thick, you can add more liquid to reach your desired thickness.

5. Taste the smoothie and adjust sweetness if necessary. You can add honey or agave syrup to sweeten, but this step is optional as the natural sweetness from the fruits may be sufficient.

6. Once the minty green smoothie reaches the desired consistency and taste, pour it into glasses.

7. Garnish with a sprig of fresh mint or a slice of cucumber for a decorative touch.

Coriander-Crusted Salmon

Ingredients:

- 4 salmon filets
- 2 tablespoons fresh coriander, finely chopped
- 1 tablespoon ground coriander
- 1 teaspoon ground cumin
- 1 teaspoon paprika
- 1 teaspoon garlic powder
- 1 teaspoon onion powder
- Salt and pepper to taste
- 2 tablespoons olive oil
- Lemon wedges for serving

Instructions:

1. Preheat your oven to 400°F (200°C).

2. In a small bowl, combine fresh coriander, ground coriander, ground cumin, paprika, garlic powder, onion powder, salt, and pepper to create the spice rub.

3. Pat the salmon filets dry with a paper towel.

4. Rub the spice mixture evenly over both sides of each salmon filet, pressing the spices onto the surface of the fish.

5. Heat olive oil in an oven-safe skillet over medium-high heat.

6. Once the oil is hot, place the salmon filets in the skillet, skin side down. Sear for 2-3 minutes until the skin is crispy and golden.

7. Carefully flip the salmon filets using a spatula.

8. Transfer the skillet to the preheated oven and bake for 8-10 minutes or until the salmon is cooked through and flakes easily with a fork.

9. Remove the skillet from the oven and let the salmon rest for a couple of minutes.

10. Serve the coriander-crusted salmon hot, garnished with lemon wedges for a burst of citrus flavor.

Oregano-Infused Quinoa Salad

Ingredients:

- 1 cup quinoa, rinsed
- 2 cups water or vegetable broth
- 1 red bell pepper, diced
- 1 cucumber, diced
- 1 cup cherry tomatoes, halved
- 1/2 red onion, finely chopped
- 1/4 cup black olives, sliced
- Feta cheese, crumbled (optional)
- Fresh oregano leaves, chopped

- 1/4 cup extra-virgin olive oil

- 2 tablespoons red wine vinegar

- 1 teaspoon Dijon mustard

- Salt and pepper to taste

- Lemon wedges for serving

Instructions:

1. In a medium saucepan, combine quinoa and water or vegetable broth. Bring to a boil, then reduce heat to low, cover, and simmer for 15-20 minutes or until the quinoa is cooked and liquid is absorbed. Fluff with a fork and let it cool.

2. In a large mixing bowl, combine the cooked quinoa, diced red bell pepper, cucumber, cherry tomatoes, chopped red onion, and black olives.

3. In a small bowl, whisk together olive oil, red wine vinegar, Dijon mustard, salt, and pepper to create the dressing.

4. Pour the dressing over the quinoa and vegetable mixture. Toss gently to coat the ingredients evenly.

5. Add fresh oregano leaves to the salad and toss again.

6. If using, sprinkle crumbled feta cheese over the salad for added creaminess.

7. Refrigerate the oregano-infused quinoa salad for at least 30 minutes to allow the flavors to meld.

8. Before serving, give the salad a final toss and adjust the seasoning if necessary.

9. Serve chilled, garnished with additional fresh oregano leaves and lemon wedges on the side.

Thyme-Roasted Sweet Potatoes

Ingredients:

- 3 large sweet potatoes, peeled and cut into cubes
- 3 tablespoons olive oil
- 1 tablespoon fresh thyme leaves
- 1 teaspoon garlic powder
- 1 teaspoon paprika
- Salt and pepper to taste

Instructions:

1. Preheat your oven to 400°F (200°C).

2. In a large mixing bowl, combine the sweet potato cubes with olive oil, fresh thyme leaves, garlic powder, paprika, salt, and pepper. Toss the sweet potatoes until they are evenly coated with the seasoning.

3. Spread the seasoned sweet potatoes in a single layer on a baking sheet. Make sure not to overcrowd the pan to ensure even roasting.

4. Roast the sweet potatoes in the preheated oven for 25-30 minutes or until they are tender and caramelized, tossing them halfway through the cooking time for even roasting.

5. Once the sweet potatoes are done, remove them from the oven and let them cool slightly before serving.

6. Garnish with additional fresh thyme leaves for a burst of herbal flavor.

Sage and Lemon Tilapia

Ingredients:

- 4 tilapia filets
- 2 tablespoons olive oil
- Zest and juice of 1 lemon
- 2 tablespoons fresh sage leaves, chopped
- 2 cloves garlic, minced
- Salt and pepper to taste
- 1/4 cup all-purpose flour (for dredging)
- 2 tablespoons unsalted butter
- Lemon wedges for serving

Instructions:

1. Pat the tilapia filets dry with a paper towel.

2. In a shallow dish, combine the flour with salt and pepper. Dredge each tilapia filet in the flour mixture, shaking off any excess.

3. In a large skillet, heat olive oil over medium-high heat.

4. Add the floured tilapia filets to the skillet and cook for 3-4 minutes per side or until golden brown and cooked through.

5. While the tilapia is cooking, in a small bowl, mix together lemon zest, lemon juice, chopped sage, and minced garlic.

6. Once the tilapia filets are cooked, reduce the heat to low and add the butter to the skillet.

7. Pour the lemon and sage mixture over the tilapia filets. Spoon some of the melted butter over the filets for added flavor.

8. Cook for an additional 1-2 minutes, allowing the flavors to meld.

9. Serve the sage and lemon tilapia hot, garnished with additional fresh sage leaves and lemon wedges on the side.

Parsley and Walnut Pesto Pasta

Ingredients:

- 8 ounces (about 225g) of your favorite pasta
- 1 cup fresh parsley leaves, packed
- 1/2 cup walnuts, toasted
- 1/2 cup grated Parmesan cheese
- 2 cloves garlic, peeled
- 1/2 cup extra-virgin olive oil
- 1 tablespoon fresh lemon juice
- Salt and pepper to taste
- Optional: Red pepper flakes for a hint of spice
- Additional grated Parmesan for serving

Instructions:

1. Cook the pasta according to package instructions in a large pot of salted boiling water. Drain and set aside.

2. In a food processor, combine fresh parsley, toasted walnuts, grated Parmesan, and peeled garlic.

3. Pulse the ingredients until they are finely chopped.

4. With the food processor running, slowly pour in the olive oil in a steady stream until the mixture becomes a smooth paste.

5. Add fresh lemon juice, salt, and pepper to the pesto. Optionally, you can add red pepper flakes for a bit of heat.

6. Taste the pesto and adjust the seasoning if needed.

7. In a large mixing bowl, toss the cooked pasta with the parsley and walnut pesto until the pasta is evenly coated.

8. Serve the parsley and walnut pesto pasta hot, garnished with additional grated Parmesan.

Dill and Yogurt Dressing

Ingredients:
- 1 cup plain Greek yogurt
- 2 tablespoons fresh dill, finely chopped
- 1 tablespoon lemon juice
- 1 clove garlic, minced
- 1 tablespoon extra-virgin olive oil
- Salt and pepper to taste

Instructions:
1. In a mixing bowl, combine plain Greek yogurt, finely chopped fresh dill, minced garlic, and lemon juice.

2. Whisk the ingredients together until well combined.

3. Gradually drizzle in the olive oil while whisking continuously to emulsify the dressing.

4. Season the dill and yogurt dressing with salt and pepper to taste.

5. Taste the dressing and adjust the lemon juice, salt, or pepper if needed to achieve your desired flavor.

6. If time allows, refrigerate the dressing for at least 30 minutes before serving to allow the flavors to meld.

7. Stir the dressing before using and serve over salads, grilled vegetables, or as a flavorful dip.

"I am the architect of my
health, and I build a
foundation of well-being."

"I am on the path to
recovery, and I embrace
each moment as a step
forward."

CONCLUSION

In conclusion, the "Lymphoma Diet Cookbook" is a valuable resource for achieving well-being through immune-boosting meals customized to lymphoma management and recovery. This cookbook inspires individuals on their road to healthier living amidst lymphoma obstacles by embracing a culinary approach that prioritizes nutrition. The meticulously crafted recipes not only satisfy the palate but also help to general well-being, highlighting the symbiotic relationship between diet and immune system strength.

The cookbook strives to improve the body's resilience through the intentional inclusion of nutrient-dense ingredients, offering critical support during the complicated and nuanced experience of managing lymphoma. It aims to make the nutritional portion of lymphoma control an accessible and enjoyable part of daily living by fostering a balance of nourishment and flavor.

As we end the book, let us remember that each meal prepared has the ability to improve one's overall health and recuperation.

These recipes are more than just a collection of ingredients; they are a commitment to well-being, a celebration of life, and a tool for boosting the body's natural defenses.

May this cookbook serve as a companion and guide, encouraging a holistic approach to health, and may the wonderful meals it inspires bring comfort and strength to people dealing with lymphoma. Here's to unleashing the power of nutritious, immune-boosting cuisine to create a healthier, tastier, and more vibrant future.

HAPPY COOKING!

LYMPHOMA DIET WEEKLY MEAL PLANNER

Meal Plan
for a week

Week:...............................

	BREAKFAST	LUNCH	DINNER	SNACKS
MON				
TUE				
WED				
THU				
FRI				
SAT				
SUN				

Shopping list

Notes:

Meal Plan
for a week

Week:.................................

	BREAKFAST	LUNCH	DINNER	SNACKS
MON				
TUE				
WED				
THU				
FRI				
SAT				
SUN				

Shopping list

______________________ ______________________
______________________ ______________________
______________________ ______________________
______________________ ______________________
______________________ ______________________

Notes:

Meal Plan
for a week

Week:..............................

	BREAKFAST	LUNCH	DINNER	SNACKS
MON				
TUE				
WED				
THU				
FRI				
SAT				
SUN				

Shopping list

Notes:

Meal Plan
for a week

Week:..................................

	BREAKFAST	LUNCH	DINNER	SNACKS
MON				
TUE				
WED				
THU				
FRI				
SAT				
SUN				

Shopping list

________________ ________________

________________ ________________

________________ ________________

________________ ________________

________________ ________________

Notes:

Meal Plan

for a week

Week:...................................

	BREAKFAST	LUNCH	DINNER	SNACKS
MON				
TUE				
WED				
THU				
FRI				
SAT				
SUN				

Shopping list

Notes:

Meal Plan

for a week

Week:..................................

	BREAKFAST	LUNCH	DINNER	SNACKS
MON				
TUE				
WED				
THU				
FRI				
SAT				
SUN				

Shopping list

Notes:

Meal Plan
for a week

Week:...............................

	BREAKFAST	LUNCH	DINNER	SNACKS
MON				
TUE				
WED				
THU				
FRI				
SAT				
SUN				

Shopping list

Notes:

Meal Plan
for a week

Week:...............................

	BREAKFAST	LUNCH	DINNER	SNACKS
MON				
TUE				
WED				
THU				
FRI				
SAT				
SUN				

Shopping list

Notes:

Meal Plan
for a week

Week:...............................

	BREAKFAST	LUNCH	DINNER	SNACKS
MON				
TUE				
WED				
THU				
FRI				
SAT				
SUN				

Shopping list

Notes:

Meal Plan
for a week

Week:................................

	BREAKFAST	LUNCH	DINNER	SNACKS
MON				
TUE				
WED				
THU				
FRI				
SAT				
SUN				

Shopping list

_______________________   _______________________

_______________________   _______________________

_______________________   _______________________

_______________________   _______________________

_______________________   _______________________

Notes: